Contents

Introduction

Hypertension is one of the major risk factors for coronary heart disease (CHD), cerebrovascular accident (CVA), chronic renal failure (CRF), and congestive heart failure (CHF) in the United States. CHD is the leading cause of death in the United States, accounting for more than 750,000 deaths per year (one death per minute).[1–3]

Hypertension is part of a heterogeneous condition that is best described as an *atherosclerotic syndrome* or *hypertension syndrome* with genetic and acquired structural and metabolic disorders, including the following:[4,5,147]

1. Dyslipidemia
2. Insulin resistance and impaired glucose tolerance
3. Central obesity
4. Endocrine changes (SNS, RAAS)
5. Renal function abnormalities (sodium, water, uric acid, protein load excretion, microalbuminuria)
6. Abnormalities of vascular and cardiac smooth muscle structure and function (arterial compliance) (LVH)
7. Membranopathy and abnormal cellular cation transport
8. Abnormalities of coagulation factors
9. Endothelial dysfunction

The *primary goal* in the treatment of hypertension is not simply to reduce intra-arterial pressure, but to treat the hypertension syndrome optimally. Ideally the optimal treatment should maximize reduction in *all* end-organ damage, including CHF, CHD, CVA, CRF, left ventricular hypertrophy (LVH), and myocardial infarction (MI).

Recent advances in our understanding of the physiology and patho-physiology of the blood vessel show that its endothelial function plays an important role in end-organ damage. Attention must be directed at promoting **VASCULAR HEALTH** in order to achieve optimal reduction in end-organ damage.

Rethink Treatment
Hypertension is a Disease of Blood Vessels

Vascular Biology is Altered
(Structural and Functional)

Target the Vasculature
- Risk Factors (Traditional)
- Risk Factors (Nontraditional—Vascular Biology)

↓

Target Organs—Optimal Treatment

■ The Blood Vessel is an Organ
- Largest Organ in the Body
- 5 × Heart in Mass
- 6 Tennis Courts in Area

The vessel wall is an active, integrated organ composed of endothelial, smooth muscle and fibroblast cells coupled to each other in a complex autocrine-paracrine set of interactions.

The Vascular System Regulates Vascular Health and Tone Through Chronic Active Balance Between:

Vasoconstrictors   Vasodilators
Growth Promoters   Growth Inhibitors

Vascular Tone
Vascular Health (Damage)

The Blood Vessel Structure

- Serosa
- Muscularis
- Endothelium

Structural and functional changes may cause dysfunction leading to vascular damage and target organ damage.

Endothelial Dysfunction:

1. Vasospasm (vasoconstriction vs. vasodilation)
2. Thrombosis (procoagulant vs. anticoagulant)
3. Atherosclerosis (proinflammatory vs. anti-inflammatory)
4. Restenosis (growth promotion vs. inhibition)

Structural Dysfunction:

1. Vascular hypertrophy
2. Vascular hyperplasia
3. Vascular polyploidy

Functional Endothelium

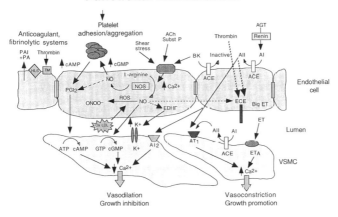

The diagram above illustrates the complexity of the processes mediated by the endothelium in carrying out its various regulatory functions. The vasorelaxant substances nitrous oxide (NO), prostacyclin, and endothelium-derived hyperpolarizing factor (EDHF) released by the endothelium promote vasodilation and inhibit growth of vascular smooth muscle cells. Angiotensin II and endothelin are potent vasoconstrictors and growth-promoting factors released from the endothelium. Bradykinin, through a receptor-mediated mechanism, stimulates release of NO. Increased expression of ACE in the endothelium increases production of angiotensin II and degradation of bradykinin, leading to decreased synthesis/release of NO from the endothelium. NO prevents platelet adhesion/aggregation and mediates synthesis of tissue plasminogen activator (t-PA), whereas angiotensin II promotes platelet aggregation and formation of plasminogen activator inhibitor (PAI-1).

Vascular Functions of Endothelium

- Maintain tone and structure
- Regulate cell growth
- Regulate thrombotic and fibrinolytic properties
- Mediate inflammatory and immune mechanisms
- Regulate leukocyte and platelet adhesion to surface
- Modulate oxidation (metabolic activity)
- Regulate permeability

Endothelial Dysfunction

Definition*

- Injury or activation of the endothelial cell leads to altered endothelial function that may promote disease.
- The dysfunctional state may be characterized by numerous features such as an imbalance between endothelium-derived relaxing and contracting factors or growth-promoting factors.

Pathophysiologic Consequences*

Macromolecular barrier disruption

↓

Increased vessel permeability

↓

Physiologic clearance mechanisms overwhelmed

↓

LDL oxidation and initiation of atherosclerosis

Hypothesis

- Normal endothelium maintains balance between relaxant and constrictive factors

- Endothelial dysfunction promotes vasoactive substance imbalance
  ↓ No
  ↑ tissue ACE
  ↑ AII

*From Lüscher TF: J Myocard Ischemia 7(Suppl 1):15–20, 1995.

Treatment of Impaired Endothelial Function

- Cholesterol lowering
- Antioxidan therapy
- Hormone replacement therapy
- L-arginine supplementation
- ACE inhibition
- Others
  Antiogensin I blockade
  Calcium blocker therapy
  Omega-3 fatty acid supplementation
  Exercise training (shear stress)
  Improve insulin resistance

Endothelial Dysfunction and Atherosclerotic Vascular Disease (Clinical Events)

- Endothelial dysfunction
- ↑ Permeability
- ↓ Antithrombotic and fibrinolytic activity
- Induction of adhesion molecules
- ↓ Vasodilator function
- Inactivation fo EDRF (oxygen free radicals)

- Vascular/atheroscelerotic effects
- LDL or blood-borne mitogen penetration to subendothelium
- ↑ Thrombosis
- ↓ Fibrinolysis
- Recruit macrophages into vascular wall
- ↓ Antioproliferative activity
- ↑ Smooth muscle cell proliferation

Estrogens and Vascular Function

- Receptor mediated
  - ↑ Endothelial NO
  - ↑ Vasodilation
  - ↓ LDL penetration
- Antioxidant nonreceptor effect

Oral therapy may result in different effects than transdermal therapy.

Antihypertensive drug therapy must recognize these challenges and concepts. *Individualization of treatment* is recommended based on the *subsets of hypertension approach.*[5] This is a logical and tailored selection of drug treatment based on:

1. Pathophysiology and vascular biology
2. Hemodynamics
3. Risk factor reduction and end-organ damage reduction
4. Concomitant medical diseases or problems
5. Demographics
6. Quality of life and adverse effects of treatment
7. Compliance with therapy
8. Total health care cost

This tenth edition of the *Handbook of Antihypertensive Therapy* has been vastly expanded and updated to incorporate these new concepts, changes in philosophy, clinical information, clinical trials, and new antihypertensive drugs and drug delivery systems. There is much controversy about hypertension treatments, and large-scale clinical trials comparing the older antihypertensive drug regimens with newer agents have been completed and many others are in progress. The recent Systolic Hypertension Trial in Europe (SYST-EUR), Shanghai Trial of Nifedipine in the Elderly (STONE), Systolic Hypertension in China (SYST-CHINA), Hypertension Optimal Treatment (HOT), and the Chen-Du Nifedipine Trial have documented significant reductions in cardiovascular and cerebrovascular morbidity and mortality with calcium channel blockers. The Captopril Prevention Project (CAPPP) showed that angiotensin-converting enzyme inhibitors reduce cardiovascular morbidity and mortality in hypertensive patients equal to conventional therapy. The Heart Outcomes Evaluation Study (HOPE) showed that ACEI reduced cardiovascular death in a high-risk nonhypertensive population. The treatment of the hypertensive patient with diabetes mellitus has now been shown in both SYST-EUR and CAPPP to be better with calcium channel blockers or angiotensin-converting enzyme inhibitors than with conventional diuretic or beta blocker therapy in reducing cardiovascular morbidity and mortality. The Swedish Trial in Old Patients–2 (STOP-2) showed that calcium blockers or ACEI are equal to conventional therapy in reducing cardiovascular morridity and mortality. New data on angiotensin-converting enzyme inhibitors and angiotension receptor blockers in cardiac disease (congestive heart failure, myocardial infarction) are positive as well. No single antihypertensive drug can meet every need in all hypertensive patients. Fortunately, the armamentarium is large and rapidly growing.

Acknowledgement: Thanks to Dr. Jordan Asher for his review of the manuscript for this edition.

Mark C. Houston, MD, FACP
ASH Specialist in Clinical Hypertension
Associate Clinical Professor of Medicine
Vanderbilt University School of Medicine

Director, Hypertension Institute
St. Thomas Medical Group
St. Thomas Hospital and Health Services
Nashville, Tennessee

Abbreviations

Ang-II	angiotensin II
ACE	angiotensin-converting enzyme
AV	atrioventricular
ARB	angiotensin II receptor blocker
BP	blood pressure
BUN	blood urea nitrogen
CHD	coronary heart disease
CHF	congestive heart failure
CO	cardiac output
CRF	chronic renal failure
CVA	cerebrovascular accident
DBP	diastolic blood pressure
DHEAS	dehydroepiandrosterone sulfate
DHP	dihydropyridine
EPI	epinephrine
GFR	glomerular filtration rate
GITS	gastrointestinal therapeutic system
HCTZ	hydrochlorothiazide
HDL	high-density lipoprotein
HR	heart rate
IBW	ideal body weight
IGCP	intraglomerular capillary pressure
ISA	intrinsic sympathomimetic activity
IVP	intravenous pyelogram (pyelography)
LDL	low-density lipoprotein
Lp(a)	lipoprotein A
LVFP	left ventricular filling pressure
LVH	left ventricular hypertrophy
MAO	monoamine oxidase
MAP	mean arterial pressure
MI	myocardial infarction
MIBG	metaiodobenzylguanidine
MRI	magnetic resonance imaging
MSA	membrane-stabilizing activity
NE	norepinephrine
NPI	neuro-peptidase inhibitors

NSAIDs	nonsteroidal anti-inflammatory drugs
PET	positron emission tomography
PFTs	pulmonary function tests
PIH	pregnancy-induced hypertension
PRA	plasma renin activity
PWP	pulmonary wedge pressure
RAAS	renin-angtotensin-aldosterone
RBC	red blood cell
RBF	renal blood flow
RPF	renal plasma flow
RVR	renal vascular resistance
SBP	systolic blood pressure
SNS	sympathetic nervous system
SV	stroke volume
SVR	systemic vascular resistance
TPA	tissue plasminogen activator
UTI	urinary tract infection
VLDL	very-low-density lipoprotein
VMA	vanillylmandelic acid

Hypothesis: Essential Hypertension and End-Organ Damage

The primary goal in the treatment of essential hypertension is to prevent and reduce *all* end-organ damage, not simply to reduce blood pressure (BP). Hypertension is associated with an increased risk of cerebrovascular, cardiovascular, and renal morbidity and mortality. Pharmacologic therapy has reduced some, but not all, of these complications. To achieve optimal decreases in morbidity and mortality in hypertensive-related diseases, the overall impact of antihypertensive drug therapy on the pathogenesis of damage to each end organ must be considered.

Although a higher percentage of deaths occurs in patients with diastolic blood pressure (DBP) ≥105 mm Hg, patients with DBP ≤105 mm Hg account for more deaths. The majority of patients with hypertension have the mild form. The risks of therapy versus the benefits of therapy are particularly critical in this group. Pharmacologic therapy of mild to moderate hypertension (DBP ≤110 mm Hg) has reduced the complications of most pressure-related (arteriolar) damage, such as CVA, CHF, and some cases of CRF, but the atherosclerotic complications (CHD, angina, MI, and sudden death) have not been reduced to the extent predicted by the degree of BP reduction in those prospective clinical trials in which diuretics and beta-blockers were the primary antihypertensive drugs used.[4] The role of beta blocker monotherapy in reducing CHD in the elderly has been questioned.[130] In addition, the indiscriminate use of diuretics, especially in young hypertensives, may be associated with a higher incidence of renal cell carcinoma and/or progressive renal insufficiency.[90,148]

A more sophisticated and pathophysiologically oriented pharmacologic approach based on our knowledge of vascular biology, endothelial dysfunction, and the complex interplay of the component of the *hypertension/atherosclerotic syndrome* is needed. The newer drugs (CCD, ACEI, ARB) appear to offer some distinct advantages in both surrogate end points and target organ damage compared to older drugs (diuretics, BB).

Hypertension in the United States and Classification

1. Approximately 50–60 million people in the United States have hypertension—BP reading greater than 140/90 mm Hg.[6] Only 27% of this population controls their hypertension according to NHANES III (Table 11).

2. Stage 1 (mild) of elevated BP (DBP <90–99 mm Hg) is the most common form of high BP in adults. Other stages of elevated BP are as follows: stage 2 (moderate, DBP 100–109 mm Hg), stage 3 (severe, DBP 110–119 mm Hg), and stage 4 (very severe, DBP ≥120 mm Hg).[6]

3. Prevalence rates: highest in African-Americans, men, and elderly. African-Americans have the greatest morbidity and mortality.[4]

4. Hypertension occurs in approximately 60% of non-Hispanic whites, 70% of non-Hispanic blacks, and 61% of Mexican-Americans aged 60 years or older.[6]

5. A large proportion (60%) of the excess mortality, disability, and morbidity attributable to hypertension occurs among those with stage 1 of the disease.[6]

6. Hypertension is the most common medical problem seen by U.S. physicians, accounting for more office visits and prescriptions than any other disease.[4]

7. In the United States and other industrialized societies, BP increases with age.[4]

8. SBP and wide pulse pressure (PP) correlate with target organ damage (TOD) better than DBP.

9. The 1997 Joint National Committee report (JNC VI) proposed the following classification of the degree of hypertension and risk stratification for treatment.[116]

Classification of Blood Pressure for Adults Aged 18 Years and Older

Category	Blood Pressure, mm Hg		
	Systolic		Diastolic
Optimal†	<120	and	<80
Normal	<130	and	<85
High-normal	130–139	or	85–89
Hypertension			
Stage 1 (mild)	140–159	or	90–99
Stage 2 (moderate)	160–179	or	100–109
Stage 3 (severe)	≥ 180	or	N ≥ 110

10. Risk Stratification and Treatment*

Blood Pressure Stages (mmHg)	Risk Group A (No Risk Factors No TOD/CCD)†	Risk Group B (At least 1 Risk Factor, Not Including Diabetes; No TOD/CCD	Risk Group C (TOD/CCD and/or Diabetes, With or Without Other Risk Factors)
High–normal (130–139/ 85–89)	Lifestyle modification	Lifestyle modification	Drug therapy§
Stage 1 (140–159/ 90–99)	Lifestyle modification (up to 12 months)	Lifestyle modification‡ (up to 6 months)	Drug therapy
Stages 2 and 3 (> 160/> 100)	Drug therapy	Drug therapy	Drug therapy

*Lifestyle modification should be adjunctive therapy for all patients recommended for pharmacologic therapy.
† TOD/CCD indicates target organ disease/clinical cardiovascular disease.
‡For patients with multiple risk factors, clinicians should consider drugs as initial therapy plus lifestyle modifications.
§ For those with heart failure, renal insufficiency, or diabetes.

11. Components of Cardiovascular Risk Stratification in Patients with Hypertension*

Major Risk Factors

Smoking

Dyslipidemia

Diabetes mellitus

Age older than 60 years

Sex (men and postmenopausal women)

Family history of cardiovascular disease:
women under age 65 or men under age 55

Target Organ Damage/Clinical Cardiovascular Disease

Heart diseases
- Left ventricular hypertrophy
- Angina/prior myocardial infarction
- Prior coronary revascularization
- Heart failure

Stroke or transient ischemic attack

Nephropathy

Peripheral arterial disease

Retinopathy

Trends in the Prevalence, Awareness, Treatment, and Control of High Blood Pressure in Adults in the U.S. 1976–1994*

Percent	NHANES II 1976–1980	NHANES II (Phase 1) 1988–1991	NHANES III (Phase 2) 1991–1994
Awareness	51	73	68
Treated	31	55	53
Controlled	10	29	27

*Adults with hypertension (SBP > 140 mm Hg or DBP > 90 mm Hg) or taking antihypertensive medication. Age 18–74 years.
NHANES = National Health and Nutritional Examination Survey.
From Arch Intern Med 157: 2414, 1997, with permission.

---

*Tables in 9, 10, and 11 are reproduced from Joint National Committee on Prevention, Detection, Evaluation, and Treatment of High Blood Pressure: The Sixth Report of the Joint National Committee on Prevention, Detection, Evaluation, and Treatment of High Blood Pressure (JNC VI). Bethesda, MD, National Institutes of Health; National Heart, Lung, and Blood Institute; 1997. NIH publication 98-4080.

Secondary Hypertension

Cause	Signs and Symptoms	Confirmation
Oral contraceptives	Recent onset of hypertension Average 5% increase in BP after 7 years	Cessation of oral contraceptive should be followed by normalization of BP within 6 months
Licorice intoxication	Eating large amounts of licorice	Cessation of licorice intake should cause normalization of BP within 1 month
Primary aldosteronism	Muscle cramps, weakness, polyuria, hypokalemia, metabolic alkalosis	Decreased PRA, increased urinary K^+, increased aldosterone, decreased serum K^+, positive saline suppression test
Pheochromocytoma	Sustained hypertension, intermittent hypertension, headaches, sweating, palpitation, pallor, tachycardia, orthostatic hypotension	24-hr urinary or serum catecholamines, VMA, CT scan, MIBG scan, MRI scan, clonidine suppression test, PET scan, metanephrines
Hyperparathyroidism	Bone pain, constipation, fatigue	Hypercalcemia, hypophosphatemia, increased parathyroid hormone
Thyroid disease	Hyperthyroidism, hypothroidism	Free thyroxine index, free triiodothyronine index, thyroid-stimulating hormone
Acromegaly	Physical findings	Growth hormone level
Decongestants	Tachycardia, sudden increased BP	History of OTC medications

Sleep apnea	Obesity, snoring, apnea, daytime somnolence	Sleep study, arterial blood gases, PFTs
Cushing's syndrome	Moon face, central obesity, hirsutism, hypokalemia, diabetes, glucose intolerance	Increased urinary 17-hydroxycorticosteroids and 17-ketosteroids and urine and plasma cortisol, loss of diurnal variation of serum cortisol, dexamethasone suppression test
Coarctation of aorta	Headache, lower extremity claudication, leg BP 20 mm Hg lower than arm BP, reduced femoral pulse, abnormal chest x-ray	Arteriography of aorta
Renal disease	Dysuria, nocturia, hematuria, RBC casts, recurrent UTI, edema	Creatinine, BUN, urinalysis, IVP, nuclear medicine GFR, ultrasound, renal biopsy
Renovascular hypertension	Recent-onset, accelerated hypertension, abdominal bruit, DBP $\geq$110 mm Hg resistant to treatment, atherosclerotic and fibromuscular dysplasia subtypes	Arteriography, renal vein renins, PRA, nuclear medicine GFR and renogram, captopril test (captopril renal scan), renal artery Doppler scan
Miscellaneous drugs or toxins (NSAIDs, sympathomimetics, cocaine, alcohol)	Hypertension or attenuation of antihypertensive drug action	Discontinue medications; serum and urine studies

Indirect Measurement of Blood Pressure[6,7,120]

Equipment

Sphygmomanometer (anaeroid or mercury manometer)

Methodology

1. The patient should be seated for 5 minutes in a quiet, comfortable environment, with the arm free of restrictive clothing or other materials and supported at heart level. The patient should avoid exertion, temperature extremes, eating, caffeine, or smoking for 1 hour before BP measurement.
2. The observer (clinician) should be at eye level of the meniscus of the mercury column or centered in front of the gauge; avoid strained posture.
3. The appropriate cuff size should be selected. The cuff bladder should be 20% wider than the diameter of the extremity. The bladder length should be approximately twice the recommended width.
4. The deflated cuff should be placed at least 2.5 cm above the antecubital space. The cuff should fit smoothly and snugly around the arm, with the bladder centered directly over the brachial artery.
5. Palpate for the brachial pulse. To estimate systolic blood pressure (SBP), rapidly inflate the cuff until the brachial pulse can no longer be felt.
6. Place the bell of the stethoscope over the previously palpated brachial artery. Rapidly inflate the cuff to 30 mm Hg above the point at which the brachial pulse disappears; deflate the cuff at the rate of 2 to 3 mm Hg/sec.
7. Record SBP as the first Korotkoff sound and DBP as the fifth Korotkoff sound.

8. Allow 1 to 2 minutes between BP determinations.

9. BP should then be determined in the upright posture after the patient has been standing for 2 minutes. The arm should be positioned at heart level, with the forearm at the horizontal level of the fourth intercostal space.

10. On the initial visit, BP readings should be performed in both arms and in the thigh. Subsequent BP determinations should be performed in the arm with the higher reading if there is more than a 10-mm Hg discrepancy in BP reading.

Korotkoff Sounds[7]

Phase I: Marked by the first appearance of faint, clear tapping sounds, which gradually increase in intensity. *Phase I should be used as the SBP.*

Phase II: Period during which a murmur or swishing sound is heard.

Phase III: Period during which sounds are crisper and increase in intensity.

Phase IV: Period marked by the distinct, abrupt muffling of sound (soft, blowing quality is heard).

Phase V: The point at which sounds disappear. *Phase V should be used as the DBP* (except on rare occasions, e.g., aortic insufficiency).

Common Mistakes in Blood Pressure Measurement[4,7]

1. Failure to keep the person in the supine position for 5 minutes before measuring the BP.
2. Failure to keep the arm at the level of the heart.
3. If Korotkoff sounds cannot be heard, failure to *completely deflate* the cuff before determining BP and failure to wait 1 to 2 minutes before doing further determinations.
4. Observer error, because of hearing impairment, bias (preferring some digits over others), or unconscious bias toward underreading or overreading BP depending on dividing line of normal.
5. Failure to keep the eyes at the level of the mercury manometer.
6. Deflating cuff too rapidly. The cuff should be deflated at a rate of 2 to 3 mm Hg/sec.
7. Failure to use appropriate cuff size. Use of a regular adult cuff for obese persons leads to a high BP reading. Use a large adult cuff or thigh cuff for obese persons; use a child's cuff for children. The cuff should cover two thirds of the arm above the antecubital space.
8. Failure to position the cuff correctly. The cuff should be placed 2 to 3 cm above the antecubital space.
9. Failure to provide a conducive environment: comfortable room temperature and quiet surroundings free of noises and distracting stimuli.
10. Missing the heart beat during auscultation in patients with excessive bradycardia.

Hypertension-Atherosclerotic Syndrome

Hypertension is not just a disorder of increased intra-arterial pressure. Rather, it is part of a *syndrome* of commonly associated genetic or acquired (or both) metabolic and structural abnormalities, including dyslipidemia, insulin resistance (hyperinsulinemia, impaired glucose tolerance, hyperglycemia, diabetes mellitus), central or portal obesity, renal function abnormalities, abnormal vascular and cardiac smooth muscle proliferation, metabolism, hypertrophy, and hyperplasia, abnormal cellular cation transport or membranopathy, endocrine changes, coagulation abnormalities, and endothelial dysfunction. These abnormalities can lead to acceleration of arterial damage, atherosclerosis, and a greater incidence of atherosclerotic cardiovascular complications. This metabolic and structural syndrome of vascular disease exists in both treated and untreated hypertensives and in children of hypertensive parents.[147] Recognition of this concept should lead to a more rational and logical approach to the treatment of hypertension.[4,147]

Prevalence of Insulin Resistance

- 63% in type 2 diabetes
- 57% in patients with low HDL-C
- 54% in hypertriglyceridemia
- 41% in impaired glucose tolerance
- 37% in hyperuricemia
- 29% in hypertension
- 25% in hypercholesterolemia

Adapted from Bonora E, Kiechel S, Willeit J, et al: Prevalence of insulin resistance in metabolic disorders: The Bruneck Study. Diabetes. 1998;47:1643–1649.

Vascular Changes and CV Risk Factors in Borderline Hypertensives (BP 130/94 mm Hg)

	vs. Normotensives
Vascular resistance	+22%
Vessel structural changes	+11%
Total cholesterol	+8%
HDL cholesterol	−7%
Triglycerides	+42%
Insulin	+43%
Glucose	+4%
Insulin resistance	+29%

From Julius S, Jamerson K, Mejia A, et al. The association of borderline hypertension with target organ changes and higher coronary risk: Tecumseh Blood Pressure study. JAMA. 1990;264:354-358.

Nonpharmacologic Treatment of Hypertension[4,8]

Nonpharmacologic therapy should be an *initial* or *adjunctive* therapy to drug therapy. An initial trial of 3 to 6 months should be instituted in patients who have mild elevations in BP without end-organ damage. In a compliant patient, these measures can be an effective means of BP reduction. (*See JNC VI Guidelines.*)

1. *Weight reduction* (to ideal body weight [IBW]): About 60% of hypertensive patients are 20% over ideal body weight. Weight loss increases cardiac output (CO) and decreases left ventricular filling pressure (LVFP), intravascular volume, insulin levels, catecholamine levels, systemic vascular resistance (SVR), Na^+ retention, sympathetic nervous system activity, renin, and aldosterone. *See page 14.*

2. *Discontinuation of smoking:* Vasoconstriction, sympathetic nervous system activity, and norepinephrine (NE) levels are reduced.

3. *Discontinuation of caffeine:* Vasoconstriction, PRA, and NE levels are reduced.

4. *Discontinuation of alcohol:* More than one or two drinks/day, 8 oz of wine, or 24 oz of beer elevates BP, PRA, aldosterone, and cortisol.

5. *Aerobic exercise and physical training:* 30 minutes per day to 80% maximal aerobic capacity for age: heart rate (HR) = (220 − age). Avoid isometric exercises; they may elevate BP. *See page 15.*

6. *Other behavioral modifications:* Stress management, biofeedback, relaxation, psychotherapy, hypnosis, transcendental meditation.

7. *Discontinuation of concomitant medications that increase BP:*
   a. Oral contraceptives.
   b. NSAIDs: Interfere with diuretics, beta-blockers, and angiotensin-converting enzyme (ACE) inhibitors.

   c. Antihistamines/decongestants and phenylpropanola-
mine.

   d. Corticosteroids and mineralocorticoids, anabolic ster-
oids.

   e. Sympathomimetics and amphetamine-like drugs.

   f. Carbenoxolone or licorice.

   g. Tricyclic antidepressants.

   h. Monoamine oxidase (MAO) inhibitors.

   i. Ergot alkaloids.

   j. Diet pills and "energy" pills.

   k. Toxins: lead, cadmium, thallium.

8. *Assurance, patient education, frequent follow-up, and improved patient compliance.*

9. *Nutritional aspects:*

   a. Sodium restriction: 2 g/day (1000 mg = 43 mEq) low-
ers DBP about 5 mm Hg. (For salt-sensitive patients:
NE levels tend to decrease. Salt-resistant patients have
less reduction.) Decreases SVR, LVH.

   b. Potassium supplementation: 80 to 100 mEq/day (reduces SVR, renal vascular resistance (RVR), renin levels, BP, natriuresis). Also reduces incidence of CVA.

   c. Polyunsaturated-to-saturated fat ratio: >1.0, with fat
supplying 20% to 25% or less of total calories. More
monounsaturated fats.

   d. Calcium supplementation: 1000 mg/day (low renin hypertension) has lowered SBP by 3.8 mm Hg.

   e. Magnesium supplementation: 300 mg/day (controversial).

   f. Carbohydrate restriction: natriuretic effect reduces
sympathetic nervous system activity and insulin levels
(glucose, sucrose, fructose) and improves insulin sensitivity.

   g. High fiber intake (crude plant fiber): 20 g/day.

   h. Dietary amino acids: leucine.

   i. Trace minerals.

   j. Fish oils and omega-3 fatty acids.

   k. Anti-oxidant therapy.

   l. Coenzyme Q-10

   m. Mediterranean diet

Obesity

1. It is unsafe to lose over 3.3 lbs/week.
2. Body fat is more important than body weight
   Males should be < 15% body fat
   Females should be < 22% body fat
3. The number of calories needed per day to keep you at the same weight is your weight in pounds plus zero.
   i.e., 160 lbs = 1600 calories
   1600 calories is your BMR (basal metabolic rate)
4. It takes a 3500 calorie deficit to lose *one pound*.
5. If your body mass index (BMI) is over 27, you are in danger of developing *significant health problems*.

$$BMI = \frac{Weight \ (pounds)}{(Height \ in \ inches)^2} \times 703 = kg/m^2$$

6. Three major factors contribute to obesity:
   • Metabolic factors
   • Diet
   • Physical inactivity
7. Waist circumference over the values below is associated with a high risk of disease:
   Men over 40 inches
   Women over 35 inches
8. Obesity will increase the risk of morbidity and mortality from the following disease:
   • Hypertension (high blood pressure)
   • Dyslipidemia (abnormal cholesterol and fat profile)
   • Type II diabetes
   • Coronary heart disease and heart attack
   • Stroke
   • Gallbladder disease
   • Osteoarthritis
   • Sleep apnea
   • Respiratory problems
   • Cancer of breast, prostate, colon, and endometrium
9. Ideal body weight calculation:
   • Women: 100 lbs first 5 feet than 5 lbs for each additional inch
   • Men: 106 lbs first 5 feet then 6 lbs for each additional inch.

Exercise Activities and Kilocalories Used

Energy Values in Kilocalories per Hour of Selected Activities

	Weight (pounds)					
	95	**125**	**155**	**185**	**215**	**245**
Slow walking	86	114	140	168	196	222
Walking, moderate pace	172	228	280	336	392	555
Hiking	285	342	420	504	588	666
Jogging	430	570	700	840	980	1,110
Running	480	770	945	1,134	1,323	1,499
Heavy housework	194	256	315	378	441	500
Sweeping	108	142	175	210	245	278
Scrubbing	237	313	385	462	539	611
Tennis	301	399	490	588	686	777
Golf (carrying clubs)	237	313	385	462	539	611
Golf (in a cart)	151	200	245	294	343	389
Swimming (light laps)	344	456	560	672	784	888
Swimming (hard laps)	430	570	700	840	980	1,110

Exercise: The Prescription

- Aerobic exercise more than isometric
- Duration: 30–45 minutes per session/daily
    - Warmup/Condition/Cooldown
    - 300 calories expenditure
- Intensity: Percent of MHR (maximum heart rate) for age: MHR = MAC (maximum aerobic capacity)
  Mild:50–60% $\times$ (220 − age)
  Moderate:70% $\times$ (220 − age)
  Heavy:80% $\times$ (220 − age)
- Methods: Walk, run, bicycle, swim, water-jog, treadmill, Nordic Ski Track, Health Rider
- Graduated supervised exercise regimen over 6–8 weeks of cardiovascular training

Approaches to Selection of Antihypertensive Therapy

1. *Stepped-care approach:* Limited usefulness.[4,5,9]
2. *Demographic approach* (race, sex, age): Limited and selected usefulness.[10]
3. *Renin profile analysis:* Limited and selected usefulness.[11,12]
4. *Subsets of hypertension:* Individualized therapy: recommended approach.[4,5,9]
   a. Pathophysiology: Membranopathy, ion transport defects, structural factors, smooth muscle hypertrophy (vascular, cardiac, cerebral, renal), functional factors, vasoconstrictive forces, endothelial dysfunction.
   b. Hemodynamics: SVR, CO, arterial compliance, organ perfusion, BP. Select the appropriate therapy to reverse the circulatory dysregulation.
   c. End-organ damage: Reduce risk factors for *all* end-organ damage.
   d. Concomitant medical diseases and problems: Select antihypertensive medications with favorable or neutral effects.
   e. Demographics: Race, age, gender.
   f. Adverse effects of drugs and quality of life.
   g. Compliance with medication regimen.
   h. Total health care costs: Direct and indirect costs.

Hemodynamics in Hypertension

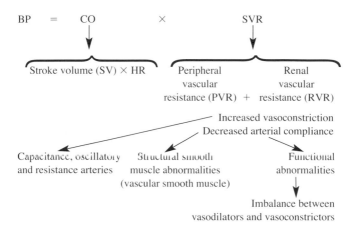

Hemodynamic Progression of Hypertension

1. *Early hypertension:* Increased CO with relative increased SVR (inappropriately increased).
2. *Established hypertension:* Decreased CO and increased SVR.
3. *Late hypertension:* Decreased CO (25%) and markedly increased SVR (25% to 30%).

All patients with essential hypertension have elevated SVR as the primary hemodynamic abnormality. Even in the uncommon case in which the CO may be transiently increased, the SVR is inappropriately elevated. Antihypertensive therapy should reverse the hemodynamic abnormalities.

Hemodynamics: Logical and Preferred Method to Reduce Blood Pressure

1. Reduce SVR.
2. Preserve CO.
3. Improve arterial compliance.
4. Maintain organ perfusion.

Achieve all the above by:

Avoiding compensatory neurohumoral reflexes, such as reflex tachycardia, salt and water overload, and reflex vasoconstrictors (NE, angiotensin II, antidiuretic hormone).

24-hour BP control.

BP control under all circumstances: rest, exercise, stress, mental function, diurnal variation.

Vascular/Arterial Compliance

1. Three vessel wall components contribute to vascular compliance
   a. Elastin: very elastic
   b. Smooth muscle: immediate elasticity
   c. Collagen: very stiff
2. Vascular compliance is composed of three arterial functions
   a. Capacitive: large conduit arteries, store blood in systole
   b. Oscillatory: small branch arteries, contribute to pressure oscillations and to reflected waves.
   c. Resistance: arterioles control blood flow and resistance function.
3. Endothelial dysfunction is first manifested in the elastin components of thin-walled arterioles (oscillatory and resistance). This raises resistance in these thin-walled arterioles prior to any effect on conduit arteries.
4. C_2-oscillatory and resistance arteriolar compliance is reduced markedly in elderly hypertensives and diabetics. Early hypertensives have reduced C_2.

    5. C_1-capacitance compliance is reduced more in isolated systolic hypertension (ISH) than in essential hypertension.

Hemodynamic Effects of Antihypertensive Drugs[4,5,9,13-30]

    1. Reduce SVR, preserve CO, and improve arterial compliance and perfusion.*
       a. Calcium channel blockers (CCB)
       b. ACE inhibitors (ACEI)
       c. Angiotensin II (Ang-II) receptor blockers (ARB)

    2. Reduce SVR, preserve CO and perfusion; effects on arterial compliance unknown.*
       a. Central alpha-agonists
       b. Alpha-blockers

    3. Reduce SVR, preserve CO and perfusion, but worsen arterial compliance.
       a. Direct vasodilators
       b. Beta-blockers with intrinsic sympathomimetic activity (ISA)
       c. Beta-blockers and alpha-blockers

    4. Reduce SVR, CO, and perfusion, and worsen arterial compliance.
       a. Diuretics
       b. Neuronal-inhibiting drugs

    5. Increase SVR and reduce CO, perfusion, and arterial compliance.
       a. Beta-blockers without ISA

---

*The best hemodynamic profile is achieved by calcium channel blockers, ACE inhibitors, Ang-II receptor antagonists, central alpha-agonists, and alpha-blockers

Hemodynamic Effects of Antihypertensive Drugs

	Diuretics	Beta-Blockers	Calcium Channel Blockers	ACE Inhibitors	Ang-II Receptor Blockers	Central Alpha-Agonists	Alpha-Blockers	Direct Vasodilators	Alpha-Blockers and Beta-Blockers	Beta-Blockers with ISA	Neuronal Inhibitors
SVR	↓/→	←	→	→	→	→	→	→	↓/→	→	→
CO	→	→	↑/→	←	←	↑	↑/←	←	↓/→	↓/→	→
SV	→	→	↑/→	←	↑	↑	↑/←	←	↓/→	↑	→
HR	→	→	↑/→	↑	↑	↓/→	→	←	↓/→	↑/←	→
RBF	←	→	→	→	→	↑/→	←	←	↓/→	↓/→	→
RVR	→	→	→	→	→	↑/→	↑/←	←	↑/←	↑	→
GFR	→	→	↓/→	→	→	↑/→	→	←	↓/→	↑	→
Cerebral blood flow	→	→	←	→	←	↑	→	←	↑	↑	↓/→
CABF	→	←/↑	←	→	→	↑/↓	↑/←	←	↑/↑	↑	←
Intravascular volume	→	→	←	→	→	↑/↓	↑/↓	←	↑/↑	↑	↑/↓
Arterial compliance	→	→	←	→	→	?	?	←	↓/→	↑	↓/↓
Perfusion	→	↑	←	→	→	→	←	→	←	←	←
LVH	↓/→	↑	→	→	→	→	→	←	→	→	→
VSM hypertrophy	←	↓/→	↑/←					←			
Exercise	↑/↓	→	↑/↑	↑	↑	↑	↑	↑	↑/↓	↑/↓	→

↓ Reduced; ↑ increased; → no change; ? unknown.
CABF = coronary artery blood flow, VSM = vascular smooth muscle

Hypertension-Related End-Organ Damage[3,31,32]

1. Cerebrovascular
   a. Cerebral infarctions: thrombotic or lacunar infarct
   b. Intracranial hemorrhage: hemorrhagic CVA
   c. Hypertensive encephalopathy
2. Cardiac
   a. CHD
      (1) Angina pectoris
      (2) MI
   b. CHF
      (1) Systolic CHF
      (2) Diastolic CHF (diastolic failure and dysfunction)
   c. LVH
   d. Sudden death
3. Renal
   a. Chronic renal insufficiency
   b. Chronic renal failure
4. Large artery disease
   a. Carotid artery stenosis and obstruction
   b. Lower extremity arterial disease or peripheral vascular disease and claudication
   c. Aortic aneurysm and dissection
5. Progression of hypertension; accelerated and malignant hypertension
6. Retinopathy

Life Expectancy and Blood Pressure (Man, 35 years old)[9,32]

1. | BP (mm Hg) | Life expectancy (years) |
   |:---:|:---:|
   | 120/80 | 76 |
   | 130/90 | 67½ |
   | 140/95 | 62½ |
   | 150/100 | 55 |

2. There is a positive correlation between BP level and total mortality.
3. The lower the SBP or DBP in either sex, the lower the mortality; the greater the BP, the higher the mortality.
4. For every 10-mm Hg rise in mean arterial pressure (MAP), there is a 40% rise in cardiovascular risk.
5. The higher the *pulse pressure*, the greater the morbidity and mortality.
6. SBP is a better predictor of cardiovascular and cerebrovascular morbidity and mortality than DBP.

Effects of Treatment of Hypertension[32–43]

The pharmacologic treatment of Stage I to Stage III (mild to moderate) hypertension (DBP ≤110 mm Hg) has reduced only some end-organ damage in the diuretic–beta-blocker trials.

1. BP reduction has reduced consequences of pressure-related arteriolar disease:
   a. Intracranial hemorrhage
   b. CHF, systolic CHF
   c. Progression of hypertension: accelerated and malignant
   d. Retinopathy
   e. Aortic aneurysm and dissection
   f. Hypertensive encephalopathy
2. BP reduction has *not* achieved expected reduction in the diuretic and beta-blocker trials in:
   a. Cerebral infarction
   b. LVH
   c. Diastolic CHF
   d. Chronic renal insufficiency and failure
3. BP reduction has *not* reduced consequences of atherosclerotic-related diseases to the predicted extent in diuretic and beta-blocker trials in:
   a. CHD
   b. Angina pectoris
   c. MI
   d. Sudden death
   e. Larger artery disease: carotid, lower extremities

Beta-blocker monotherapy does *not* reduce CHD or MI in the elderly. However, the recent STONE, SYST-EUR, SYST-CHINA, HOT, STOP-2, and CHEN-DU prospective clinical trials have shown significant reductions in cardiovascular and cerebrovascular morbidity and mortality with the calcium channel blockers. CAPP, STOP-2, and HOPE have demonstrated significant reductions in CV disease as well with ACEI.

Selected Controlled, Randomized Clinical Trials with Diuretics and Beta-Blockers in Mild to Moderate Hypertension and Coronary Heart Disease, 1979–1992

Trial (Date)	Blind	No. of Patients	Initial DBP (mm Hg)	Treatment	Mean Duration (years)	CHD Incidence
HDFP (1979)[33]	No	10,940	90–114	Referred care vs. stepped care	5	Decreased
VA Cooperative (1970)[34]	Double	380	90–114	Placebo vs. diuretics + reserpine + hydralazine	3.8	No difference
Oslo (1980)[37]	No	785	90–109	None vs. diuretics + methyldopa + propranolol	10	Increased
Australian (1980)[38]	Double	3427	95–110	Placebo vs. diuretics + methyldopa + propranolol + pindolol	4.1	No difference
MRC (1984)[39]	Single	17,354	90–109	Placebo vs. bendrofluazide or propranolol	5	No difference
MRFIT (1982)[40]	Open	8012	90–114	Thiazide diuretics	7	No difference
EWPHE (1985)[41]	Double	840	90–120	Placebo vs. thiazide diuretics + triamterene + methyldopa	4.8	No difference
MPPCD (1985)[42]	No	1203	95–110	No drug vs. pindolol + propranolol, diuretics,	5	Increased

Study	Blinding	N	BP (mmHg)	Comparison	Years	Result
USPHS (1977)[45]	Double	389	90–115	Placebo vs. diuretics + reserpine	7–10	No difference
VA-NHLBI (1978)[46]	Double	1012	85–105	Placebo vs. chlorthalidone + reserpine	1–5	No difference
IPPPSH (1972)[47]	Double	6357	100–125	No treatment vs. oxprenolol	3–5	No difference
HEP (1986)[48]	No	884	105–120	No treatment vs. atenolol + thiazide diuretics	8	No difference
HAPPHY (1987)[49]	No	6500	100–130	Diuretics vs. atenolol or metoprolol	4	No difference
MAPHY (1988)[50]	No	3234	100–130	Metoprolol vs. thiazide diuretics	5	Less in metoprolol vs. thiazides
SHEP (1991)[51]	Double	4736	SBP>160 DBP<90	Placebo vs. thiazide diuretics + beta-blockers	5	Decrease in nonfatal MI only
STOP (1991)[52]	Double	1627	105–120	Moduretic, atenolol, metoprolol, or pindolol	5	No difference

HDFP, Hypertension Detection and Follow-up Program; MRC, Medical Research Council Trial; MRFIT, Multifactorial Risk Factor Intervention Trial; EWPHE, European Working Party on Hypertension in the Elderly; MPPCD, Multifactorial Primary Prevention of Cardiovascular Diseases; USPHS, U.S. Public Health Service Trial; VA-NHLBI, Veterans Administration–National Heart, Lung, and Blood Institute; IPPPSH, International Prospective Primary Prevention Study in Hypertension; HEP, Hypertension in the Elderly; HAPPHY, Heart Attack Primary Prevention in Hypertension; MAPHY, Metoprolol Atherosclerosis Prevention in Hypertension Trial; SHEP, Systolic Hypertension In the Elderly Program; STOP, Swedish Trial In Old Patients with Hypertension.

Diuretic and Beta-Blocker Clinical Trials in Mild to Moderate Hypertension and Coronary Heart Disease: *Summary*

CHD Mortality Increase

Oslo	1980
MPPCD	1985

Sudden Death Increased (Abnormal electrocardiogram [ECG])

MRFIT	1982
HDFP	1979

CHD Mortality Decreased

HDFP	1979	
SHEP	1991	(SBP > 160)
MRC #2	1992	(diuretic group only, not beta-blocker group)
MAPHY	1988	(beta-blocker better than diuretic; no placebo)

No Difference in CHD Mortality Between Control vs. Treatment or Aggressive vs. Less Aggressive Treatment

VA Cooperative	1970
USPHS	1977
VA-NHLBI	1978
Australian	1980
MRC	1984
MRFIT	1982
EWPHE	1985
IPPPSH	1972
HEP	1986
HAPPHY	1987
STOP	1991

Clinical Hypertension Trials with Calcium Channel Blockers

1. **STONE**: Shanghai Trial of Nifedipine in the Elderly
2. **SYST-EUR**: Systolic Hypertension in Europe Trial
3. **CHEN-DU**: Nifedipine Trial
4. **SYST-CHINA**: Systolic Hypertension in China Trial
5. **HOT**: Hypertension Optimal Treatment Trial
6. **NICS-EH**: National Intervention Cooperative Study in Elderly Hypertensives

1. **STONE** (Journal of Hypertension 1996;14:1237–1245)
   - Single blind
   - 1632 men and women (Chinese)
   - Age 60–79
   - 3-year study with 30-month mean followup
   - Nifedipine tablets 10 mg (not GITS)
   - Placebo control
   - Add on treatment: Captopril or HCTZ

Number and Significance of High-Incidence Endpoints

	Original Treatment Assignment		
	Number of Events		
	Placebo	Nifedipine	Significance (p)
All events	77	32	0.0001
CV events	59	24	0.0001
Strokes	36	16	0.0030
Severe arrhythmia	13	2	0.0007
Non-CV events	18	8	0.0366
All deaths	26	15	0.0614
CV deaths	14	11	0.4870

2. **SYST–EUR** (Lancet 1997; 350:757–764)
   - Study Dates: 1990–1996, 198 centers
   - 4695 patients > 60 years (average age 70)
   - Two-thirds female
   - BP: SBP 160–219 mmHg
       DBP < 95 mmHg
   - Drugs
       Nitrendipine   10–40 mg qd
         (two-thirds on monotherapy)
       Enalapril   5–20 mg qd
       HCTZ 12.5–25 mg qd

SYST-EUR Results

	Placebo	Treatment
SBP (mm Hg)	13	23
DBP (mm Hg)	2	7

	Placebo (1000 pt. yrs)	Treatment (1000 pt. yrs)	% Reduction (p)
Total CVA	13.7	7.9	42% (.003)
Nonfatal CVA			44% (.007)
Cardiac total events	20.5	15.1	26% (0.03)
Nonfatal cardiac events			33% (0.03)
CV total	33.9	23.3	31% (.001)
CV mortality	13.5	9.8	27% (0.07)
CHF events	8.7	6.2	29% (0.12)
MI	8.0	5.5	30% (0.12)
MI deaths	2.6	1.2	56% (0.08)

Conclusions of SYST-EUR Study

1. Treatment of elderly patients with isolated systolic hypertension with nitrendipine reduces the rate of cardiovascular and cerebrovascular complications.
2. Treatment of 1000 patients for 5 years prevents 29 CVA or 53 major cardiovascular endpoints.
3. There was no increase in bleeding or cancer with nitrendipine compared with placebo.
4. Diabetic hypertensives had dramatic reductions in total mortality CV events, CVA, and coronary events on a CCB that was superior to diuretics and BB in SHEP (see pg. 57).

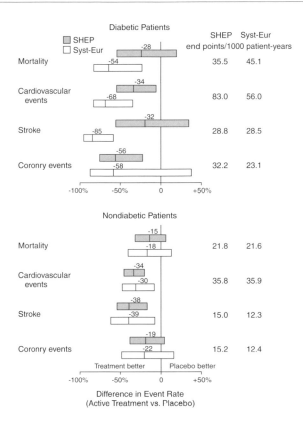

Outcomes in the Systolic Hypertension in the Elderly Program (SHEP) Trial. For these comparisons, the end points were standardized according to the definitions used in the SHEP trial. The two right-hand columns show the number of events per 1000 patient-years in the placebo groups in the two trials. The bars indicate the 95% confidence intervals. The numbers above the bars indicate the benefit of the active treatment as compared with placebo. (From Tuomilehto J, Rastenyte D, Birkenhäger W, et al: Effects of calcium-channel blockade in older patients with diabetes and systolic hypertension. N Engl J Med 1999; 340:677–684, with permission.)

3. CHEN-DU Nifedipine Trial
- 683 hypertensive patients
- Cardiovascular events at 6 years reduced from 14.0% to 5.2% (p = 0.05) in treated group

4. Systolic Hypertension in China Trial[128]

- 2400 patients over 60 with ISH
- Nitrendipine vs. placebo
  Some received captopril or HCTZ
- Goal SBP < 150 mm Hg or 20 mm Hg decrease
- Median follow-up 2 years 10 months

SYST-CHINA Results

• All cause mortality	↓ 79%
• Cardiovascular mortality	↓ 32%
• Total fatal and nonfatal cardiovascular events	↓ 37%
• Congestive heart failure	↓ 58%
• Cerebrovascular accidents	↓ 58%
• Myocardial infarction	No difference
• Fatal cancer	No difference

5. Hypertension Optimal Treatment (HOT) Trial #1

- 18,700 patients, 26 countries, age 50–80
- DBP 100–115 mm Hg
- Randomized to 3 treatment groups
  DBP ≤ 90 mm Hg → 85.2
  DBP ≤ 85 mm Hg → 83.2
  DBP ≤ 80 mm Hg → 81.1
- Felodipine   78%
  ACEI   41%
  Beta-blockers   28%
  Diuretics   22%
- ASA vs. placebo

HOT Trial #2 Results

- Lowest incidence of major CV events at DBP 82.6 mm Hg
- Optimal SBP at 138.5 mm Hg
- CV risk reduced by 30% and is lower than that observed in prospective trials using diuretics or beta-blockers (p < .05)
- Quality of Life (QOL) improved in all groups, but most in DBP < 80 mm Hg
- ASA reduced CV events by 15%, MI by 36%, but no change in CVA. Nonfatal bleeds greater, but no difference in fatal bleeds
- No increased risk of CV even down to DBP of 70 mm Hg
- CV risk reduction was even more significant in diabetic hypertensives (p <.005)

6. National Intervention Cooperative Study in Elderly Hypertensives (NICS-EH)

CCB vs. Diuretic

- 414 patients, age > 60, started 1989
- SBP 160-220 mm Hg
- DBP < 115 mm Hg
- Treatment: Nicardipine SR 20 mg bid vs. Trichlomethiazide 2 mg qd
- 5 year followup in Japan
  CCB: 172/94 mm Hg → 147/81 mm Hg
  Diuretic: 173/93 mm Hg → 147/79 mm Hg
- Results:
  Cardiovascular end points:
  CCB: 10.3%, Diuretic: 8.6%, P-value: NS
  Cardiovascular morbidity
  CCB: 27.8%, Diuretic: 26.8%, P-value: NS
  Rates per 1000 persons per year

Modified from National Intervention Cooperative Study in Elderly Hypertensives Study Group: Randomized double-blind comparison of a calcium antagnoist and a diuretic in elderly hypertensives. Hypertension 1999;34:1129-1133.

Clinical Trials in Hypertension with Angiotensin-Converting Enzyme Inhibitors: Captopril Prevention Project (CAPPP)[133]

Relative Risk of Captopril vs. Conventional Therapy

	Relative risk* (95% CI)	p	Favours captopril	Favours conventional
Primary endpoint	1.05 (0.90–1.22)	0.52		
Fatal cardiovascular events	0.77 (0.57–1.04)	0.092		
Stroke, fatal and non-fatal	1.25 (1.01–1.55)	0.044		
Myocardial infarction, fatal and non-fatal	0.96 (0.77–1.19)	0.68		
All fatal events	0.93 (0.76–1.14)	0.49		
All cardiac events	0.94 (0.83–1.06)	0.30		
Diabetes mellitus	0.86 (0.74–0.99)	0.039		

Relative Risk in Previously Untreated Patients (n = 5245)

	Relative risk* (95% CI)	p	Favours captopril	Favours conventional
Primary endpoint	0.92 (0.72–1.16)	0.47		
Fatal cardiovascular events	0.54 (0.33–0.89)	0.015		
Stroke, fatal and non-fatal	1.18 (0.84–1.65)	0.34		
Myocardial infarction, fatal and non-fatal	0.84 (0.59–1.21)	0.35		
All fatal events	0.89 (0.64–1.23)	0.48		
All cardiac events	0.93 (0.77–1.13)	0.48		
Diabetes mellitus	0.78 (0.62–0.99)	0.041		

Relative Risk in Patients with Diabetes Mellitus at Baseline (n = 572)

	Relative risk* (95% CI)	p	Favours captopril	Favours conventional
Primary endpoint	0.59 (0.38–0.91)	0.019		
Fatal cardiovascular events	0.48 (0.21–1.10)	0.085		
Stroke, fatal and non-fatal	1.02 (0.55–1.88)	0.95		
Myocardial infarction, fatal and non-fatal	0.34 (0.17–0.67)	0.002		
All fatal events	0.54 (0.31–0.96)	0.034		
All cardiac events	0.67 (0.46–0.96)	0.030		

All three charts above are reprinted with permission from Hansson L, Lindholm LH, Niskanen L, et al: Effect of angiotensin-converting enzyme inhibition compared with conventional therapy on cardiovascular morbidity and mortality in hypertension: The Captopril Prevention Project (CAPPP). Lancet. 1999;611–616.

*Adjusted for age, sex, systolic blood pressure, and previous treatment.

Heart Outcomes Prevention Evaluation Study
(HOPE)

9297 High-risk Patients Over Age 55 with:
Vascular Disease
Diabetes Mellitus + One CV Risk Factor

Ramipril	10 mg qd vs. placebo x 5 years			
Ramipril:	653 patients reached 1 endpoint	14.1%	P=<.001	
Placebo:	824 patients reached 1 endpoint	17.1%	Primary end points	

	Ramipril	Placebo	P
CV Death	6.1%	8.1%	<.001
MI	9.9%	12.2%	<.001
CVA	3.4%	4.9%	<.001
CHF	7.4%	9.4%	<.001

BP Reduced 3/2 mm Hg 40% of CVA and 25% of MI

Adapted from The Heart Outcomes Prevention Evaluation Study Investigators: Effects of angiotensin-converting-enzyme inhibitor, ramipril, on cardiovascular events in high-risk patients. New Engl J Med 2000;342:145-153.

Conventional Therapy vs. Newer Drug Therapy
Swedish Trial in Old Patients – 2 (STOP-2)

6614 Patients 70-84 years - 5 years
SBP ≥ 180 mm Hg, DBP ≥ 105 mm Hg
Diuretic or BB vs CCB or ACEI
Equal BP Reduction
CV Morbidity and Mortality was Equal

Conventional	19.8 events/1000	ACEIs	20.5 events/1000
New Drugs	19.8 events/1000	CCBs	19.2 events/1000
Last Visit:	46% on 2 Drugs		
	61-66% on Initial Drugs		
Drug Combinations:	BB +Diuretic		
	Diuretic + BB		
	CCB + BB		
	ACE + Diuretic		
Specific Drugs:	BBs: Atenolol, metoprolol, pindolol		
	Diuretics: Hydrochlorothiazide, amiloride		
	ACEIs: Enalapril, lisinopril		
	CCBs: Felodipine, isradipine		

Adapted from Hansson L, Lindholm LH, Ekbom T, et al, for the STOP-Hypertension-2 Study Group: Randomized trial of old and new antihypertensive drugs in elderly patients: Cardiovascular mortality and morbidity the Swedish Trial in Old Patients with Hypertension-2 study. Lancet 1999;354:1751-1756.

STOP-2
Relative Risk of CV Mortality and Morbidity for All Newer Drugs vs. Conventional Drugs[†]

	Relative risk* (95% CI)	p	Newer drugs better	Conventional drugs better
Cardiovascular mortality	0.99 (0.84-1.16)	0.89		
All myocardial infarction	1.04 (0.86-1.26)	0.69		
All stroke	0.89 (0.76-1.04)	0.13		
All major cardiovascular events	0.96 (0.86-1.08)	0.49		
Total mortality	1.01 (0.89-1.14)	0.92		
Frequency of diabetes mellitus	0.96 (0.75-1.23)	0.77		
Frequency of atrial fibrillation	1.09 (0.92-1.31)	0.32		
Frequency of congestive heart failure	0.95 (0.79-1.14)	0.55		

*Adjusted for age, sex, diabetes, diastotic blood pressure and smoking.
[†]Conventional drugs = atenolol, metoprolol, pindolol, hydrochlorothiazide, amiloride
  CCBs = felodipine, isradipine

STOP-2
Relative Risk of CV Mortality and Morbidity for ACE Inhibitors vs. Conventional Drugs[†]

	Relative risk* (95% CI)	p	ACE inhibitors better	Conventional drugs better
Cardiovascular mortality	1.01 (0.84-1.22)	0.89		
All myocardial infarction	0.90 (0.72-1.13)	0.38		
All stroke	0.90 (0.74-1.08)	0.24		
All major cardiovascular events	0.94 (0.82-1.07)	0.32		
Total mortality	1.02 (0.89-1.18)	0.76		
Frequency of diabetes mellitus	0.96 (0.72-1.27)	0.77		
Frequency of atrial fibrillation	1.15 (0.94-1.41)	0.18		
Frequency of congestive heart failure	0.83 (0.67-1.03)	0.095		

*Adjusted for age, sex, diabetes, diastotic blood pressure and smoking.
[†]Conventional drugs = atenolol, metoprolol, pindolol, hydrochlorothiazide, amiloride
  CCBs = felodipine, isradipine

STOP-2
Relative Risk of CV Mortality and Morbidity for
Calcium Antagonists vs. Conventional Drugs[†]

	Relative risk* (95% CI)	p	Calcium antagonists better	Conventional drugs better
Cardiovascular mortality	0.97 (0.80-1.17)	0.72		
All myocardial infarction	1.18 (0.95-1.47)	0.13		
All stroke	0.88 (0.73-1.06)	0.16		
All major cardiovascular events	0.99 (0.87-1.12)	0.85		
Total mortality	0.99 (0.86-1.15)	0.90		
Frequency of diabetes mellitus	0.97 (0.73-1.29)	0.83		
Frequency of atrial fibrillation	1.04 (0.85-1.29)	0.68		
Frequency of congestive heart failure	1.06 (0.87-1.31)	0.56		

*Adjusted for age, sex, diabetes, diastolic blood pressure and smoking.
[†]Conventional drugs = atenolol, metoprolol, pindolol, hydrochlorothiazide, amiloride
  CCBs = felodipine, isradipine

STOP-2
Relative Risk of CV Mortality and Morbidity for
ACE Inhibitors vs. Calcium Antagonists[†]

	Relative risk* (95% CI)	p	ACE inhibitors better	Calcium antagonists better
Cardiovascular mortality	1.04 (0.86-1.26)	0.67		
All myocardial infarction	0.77 (0.61-0.96)	0.018		
All stroke	1.02 (0.84-1.24)	0.84		
All major cardiovascular events	0.95 (0.83-1.08)	0.42		
Total mortality	1.03 (0.89-1.19)	0.71		
Frequency of diabetes mellitus	0.98 (0.74-1.31)	0.91		
Frequency of atrial fibrillation	1.10 (0.90-1.34)	0.37		
Frequency of congestive heart failure	0.78 (0.63-0.97)	0.025		

*Adjusted for age, sex, diabetes, diastotic blood pressure and smoking.
[†]Conventional drugs = atenolol, metoprolol, pindolol, hydrochlorothiazide, amiloride
  CCBs = felodipine, isradipine
  ACEI = enalapril, lisinopril

All five STOP-2 charts above are reprinted with permission from Hansson L, Lindholm LH, Ekbom T, et al, for the STOP-Hypertension-2 Study Group: Randomized trial of old and new antihypertensive drugs in elderly patients: Cardiovascular mortality and morbidity the Swedish Trial in Old Patients with Hypertension-2 study. Lancet 1999;354:1751-1756.

Coronary Heart Disease: Risk Factors[53–55]

1. Hypertension—SBP and DBP.*
2. Hyperlipoproteinemia:*
   a. Hypercholesterolemia: increased LDL cholesterol (especially oxidized LDL and small dense LDL);
   b. Decreased HDL cholesterol.
      (1) High HDL_2 subfraction is associated with low incidence of CHD.
      (2) HDL_3 subfraction: less CHD association.
   c. Hypertriglyceridemia: VLDL elevation (often seen with low HDL) (especially those with increased total cholesterol).
   d. Apolipoprotein A-I and A-II: low levels.
   e. Apolipoprotein B: high levels.
   f. Lipoprotein A (Lp[a]): high levels.
3. Smoking.*
4. Hyperglycemia and diabetes mellitus.
5. Insulin resistance.*
6. Family history of premature cardiovascular disease.
7. Physical inactivity (lack of aerobic exercise).*
8. LVH.*
9. Stress.
10. Type A personality (aggressive subtype).
11. Obesity (central).*
12. Male gender.
13. Hyperuricemia.*
14. Caffeine abuse (controversial).
15. Age.

---

*Factors modified by antihypertensive therapy.

Coronary Heart Disease: More Potential Risk Factors[55-67]

1. Lack of estrogen (estrogen elevates HDL_2).[56,57] (transdermal vs. oral)
2. Excessive intake of alcohol: May increase risk; however, small quantities of alcohol increase HDL_3 subfraction but are associated with decreased risk of CHD.[55,58]
3. Increased platelet adhesion or aggregation (or both) and abnormal thrombogenic potential (TPA/PAI-1 ratio).*[59,60]
4. Hemodynamic effects that alter arterial flow disturbances and induce endothelial damage, which enhances atherosclerosis (blood velocity, surfaces).*[61]
5. Renin and angiotensin II. Vasculotoxic and induce LVH¥[62,63] and endothelin.
6. Sympathetic nervous system overactivity, elevated catecholamines, vasculotoxic (NE and epinephrine [EPI] levels): Induces LVH.*[64]
7. Elevated blood viscosity.*[65]
8. Hyperinsulinemia.*[66,67]
9. Hyperfibrinogenemia* and C-reactive protein (CRP).
10. Elevated homocysteine levels.
11. Low vitamins C, A, and E levels (antioxidants).
12. Leukocytosis.
13. Corneal arcus, diagonal earlobe crease, and hairy earlobes.
14. Linoleic acid deficiency.
15. Short stature.
16. Low levels of dehydroepiandrosterone sulfate (DHEAS).
17. Nonspecific ST-T wave changes on ECG.
18. Lower socioeconomic status.
19. Increased plasma levels of rapid inhibitor of TPA.
20. Elevated serum estradiol in men.
21. Chromium deficiency.
22. Lean hypertensive men (bottom 20% of IBW).
23. Polycythemia.
24. Hypomagnesemia.[5]
25. Male pattern baldness.
26. Elevated serum creatinine.[5]
27. Microalbuminuria and proteinuria.[5]
28. Chronic tachycardia.
29. Elevated serum iron.
30. Chronic viral infections.

31. Chronic *Helicobacter pylori*—peptic ulcer disease.
32. *Chlamydia pneumoniae*
33. Chronic periodontal infection.
34. Osteoporosis at menopause.
35. Chronic cough or chronic inflammatory lung disease
36. Hypochloremia
37. Elevated intracellular adhesion molecules (ICAM-1)

*Factors modified by antihypertensive therapy.

Coronary Heart Disease Risk Factors: Influence of Diuretic and Beta-Blocker Therapy

	Diuretic (Thiazide and Thiazide-like)	Beta-Blocker (without ISA)
Hypokalemia	Yes	No
Hypomagnesemia	Yes	No
Dyslipidemia	Yes	Yes
Hypercholesterolemia	Yes	Yes or no change
Hypertriglyceridemia	Yes	Yes
Elevated LDL cholesterol	Yes	Yes or no change
Lowered HDL cholesterol	Yes or no change	Yes
Elevated apolipoprotein B	Yes	Yes
Lowered apolipoprotein A	Yes	Yes
Elevated Lp(a)	Yes	Yes
Glucose intolerance (hyperglycemia)	Yes	Yes
Insulin resistance	Yes	Yes
Hyperuricemia	Yes	Yes
Impaired aerobic exercise	Yes—minimal	Yes
LVH regression	No change	Inconsistent
Improved diastolic dysfunction	No	Inconsistent
Increased blood viscosity	Yes	No
Increased catecholamines	Yes	Yes
Increased angiotensin II	Yes	No
Potentiated arrhythmias	Yes	No
Acid-base abnormalities and other electrolyte disorders	Yes	No
Blood velocity and arterial turbulence abnormalities	Yes	No
Hyperfibrinogenemia	Yes	No
Abnormal platelet function (aggregation and adhesion)	Yes	No
Increased thrombogenic potential	Yes	No

Antihypertensive Drugs and Serum Lipids[5,68,77]

Antihypertensive Drugs with Known Unfavorable Effects on Serum Lipids

1. Diuretics: thiazides, chlorthalidone, loop diuretics, thiazide-like diuretics, metolazone
2. Beta-blockers (without ISA):
   a. Atenolol (Tenormin)
   b. Betaxolol (Kerlone)
   c. Metoprolol (Lopressor, Toprol XL)
   d. Nadolol (Corgard)
   e. Propranolol (Inderal LA)
   f. Timolol (Blocadren)
   g. Bisoprolol (Zebeta)
3. Methyldopa (Aldomet)
4. Reserpine

Antihypertensive Drugs with Potentially Favorable Effects on Serum Lipids

1. Alpha-blockers:
   a. Doxazosin (Cardura)
   b. Prazosin (Minipress)
   c. Terazosin (Hytrin)
2. Calcium channel blockers:
   a. Amlodipine (Norvasc)
   b. Diltiazem (Cardizem SR, CD, Dilacor XR, Tiazac)
   c. Felodipine (Plendil)
   d. Isradipine (DynaCirc)
   e. Nicardipine (Cardene and Cardene SR)
   f. Nifedipine (Adalat CC, Adalat Oros, Procardia XL)
   g. Verapamil (Calan SR, Isoptin SR, Verelan, Covera HS)
   h. Nisoldipine (Sular)

3. Central alpha-agonists:
   a. Clonidine (Catapres and Catapres-TTS)
   b. Guanabenz (Wytensin)
   c. Guanfacine (Tenex)

Antihypertensive Drugs with Neutral Effects on Serum Lipids

1. ACE inhibitors:
   a. Benazepril (Lotensin)
   b. Captopril (Capoten)
   c. Enalapril (Vasotec)
   d. Fosinopril (Monopril)
   e. Lisinopril (Prinivil, Zestril)
   f. Quinapril (Accupril)
   g. Ramipril (Altace)
   h. Moexidril (Univasc)
   i. Trandolapril (Mavik)
   j. Perindopril (Aceon)
2. Direct vasodilators:
   a. Hydralazine (Apresoline)
   b. Minoxidil (Loniten)
3. Beta-blockers with ISA:
   a. Acebutolol (Sectral)
   b. Penbutolol (Levatol)
   c. Pindolol (Visken)
   d. Carteolol (Cartrol)
4. Beta-blockers with alpha blocking activity:
   a. Labetalol (Trandate, Normodyne)
   b. Carvedilol (Coreg)
5. Indapamide (Lozol)
6. Angiotensin II inhibitors:
   a. Losartan (Cozaar)
   b. Valsartan (Diovan)
   c. Irbesartan (Avapro)
   d. Telmisartan (Micardis)
   e. Candesartan cilexetil (Atacand)
   f. Eprosartan (Teveten)

Serum Lipids and Antihypertensive Therapy with Diuretics and Beta-Blockers: *Summary*

1. Dose related: Higher doses of beta-blockers have more adverse effects, but even low doses of thiazide diuretics (hydrocholorothiazide [HCTZ] 12.5 mg) have adverse effects.
2. Elevations blunted but *not* prevented by:
   a. Nutritional restriction of fats and weight loss.
   b. Exercise and reduction of smoking.
3. Duration: Adverse effects persist with long-term therapy well above initial control serum lipid levels.
4. Diuretics plus beta-blockers cause additive adverse effects.
5. Thiazide and thiazide-like diuretics have similar adverse lipid effects in equipotent doses except for indapamide, which has neutral effects on lipids.
6. Beta-blockers may differ depending on several factors:
   a. Nonselective: Greatest adverse alteration in serum lipids.
   b. Cardioselective: Less adverse alteration in serum lipids.
   c. ISA: Least alteration in lipids (neutral effect).
7. Diuretic effects on serum lipids appear to be more pronounced in postmenopausal women, men, and obese patients.
8. Increase in lipids is more marked in patients with higher baseline values (average change is about 10% to 20%).
9. Abnormal lipid levels reverse to normal after cessation of therapy (takes 2 to 4 months).

Effects of Antihypertensive Drugs on Coronary Heart Disease Risk Factors[5,78–84]

	Diuretics	Indapamide	Beta-Blockers without ISA	Beta-Blockers with ISA	Labetalol
Hypertension	↓	↓	↓	↓	↓
Dyslipidemia	↑	→	↑	→	→
Glucose intolerance	↑	→	↑	↑	↑
Insulin resistance	↑	→	↑	↑	?
LVH	→/↑	↓	→	↑	↓
Exercise	→/↓	→	↓	↓	→/↓
Potassium	↓	↓*	→/↑	→	→
Magnesium	↓	↓*	→	→	→
Uric acid	↑	↑*	↑	↑	↑
Blood viscosity	↑	→	→	→	→
Blood velocity	→/↑	→	↓	→	→
Catecholamines	↑	↓	↑	↑	→
Angiotensin II	↑	→	↓	→	↓
Arrhythmia potential	↑	→	↓	→/↑	→
Fibrinogen	↑	→	?	?	?
Platelet function	↑	↓	→/↓	?	?
Thrombogenic potential	↑	↓	?	?	?
Antiatherogenic	→	→	↑†	?	?
CHD relative risk ratio	16:18	3:18	6:18	7:18	3:18

*Minimal.
†Animal studies.
‡Animal and human studies.
↓, Reduced; ↑, increased; →, no change; ?, unknown.

Continues on opposite page

Guane-thidine, Guanadrel	Central Alpha-Agonists	Methyl-dopa	Direct Vasodilators	Alpha-Blockers	Ang-II Inhibitors + ACE Inhibitors	Calcium Blockers	Reserpine
↓	↓	↓	↓	↓	↓	↓	↓
→	↓	↑	→	↓	→	↓	↑
→	↓	→	⇉	↓	↓	↓	⇉
?	↓	→	→	↓	↓	→/↓	?
↓	↓	↓	↑	↓	↓	↓	↓
↓	→	→	→	→	→	→	↓
→	→	→	→	→	↑	→	→
→	→	→	→	→	→/↑	→	→
→	→/↓	→/↓	→	→	↓	→/↓	→
→	→	→	↓	↓	→	?	?
→	↓	↑	↑	↓	↓	↓	↓
↓	↓	↓	↑	→/↓	↓	↓	↓
↑	↓	↓	↑	→/↓	↓	↓	↓
↑	↓	↓	↑	→	↓	↓	↑
?	?	?	?	↓	?	?	?
?	↓	→	?	?	↓	↓	?
?	?	?	?	?	?	↓	?
↑	?	?	?	?	↓[†]	↓[‡]	↑[†]
3:18	0:18	2:18	5:18	0:18	0:18	0:18	3:18

Antihypertensive Drugs and Coronary Heart Disease Risk Factors: *Summary*

Favorable Effects (0:18 CHD Relative Risk Ratio)

1. *Calcium channel blockers:*
   a. Amlodipine (Norvasc)
   b. Diltiazem (Cardizem SR and CD, Dilacor XR, Tiazac)
   c. Felodipine (Plendil)
   d. Isradipine (DynaCirc)
   e. Nicardipine (Cardene, Cardene SR)
   f. Nifedipine (Adalat CC, Adalat Oros, Procardia XL)
   g. Verapamil (Calan SR, Isoptin SR, Verelan, Covera HS)
   h. Nisoldipine (Sular)
2. *Alpha-blockers:*
   a. Doxazosin (Cardura)
   b. Prazosin (Minipress)
   c. Terazosin (Hytrin)
3. *Central alpha-agonists:*
   a. Clonidine (Catapres and Catapres-TTS)
   b. Guanabenz (Wytensin)
   c. Guanfacine (Tenex)
4. *ACE inhibitors:*
   a. Benazepril (Lotensin)
   b. Captopril (Capoten)
   c. Enalapril (Vasotec)
   d. Fosinopril (Monopril)
   e. Lisinopril (Prinivil, Zestril)
   f. Quinapril (Accupril)
   g. Ramipril (Altace)
   h. Moexipril (Univasc)
   i. Trandolapril (Mavik)
   j. Perindopril (Aceon)
5. *Angiotensin II blockers:*
   a. Losartan (Cozaar)
   b. Valsartan (Diovan)
   c. Irbesartan (Avapro)
   d. Telmisartan (Micardis)
   e. Candesartan cilexetil (Atacand)
   f. Eprosartan (Teveten)

Neutral Effects (0–5:18 CHD Relative Risk Ratio)

1. *Diuretics (selected):*
   a. Amiloride (Midamor)
   b. Indapamide (Lozol)
   c. Spironolactone (Aldactone)
   d. Triamterene (Dyrenium)
2. *Direct vasodilators:*
   a. Hydralazine (Apresoline)
   b. Minoxidil (Loniten)
3. *Central alpha-agonist:*
   a. Methyldopa (Aldomet)
4. *Alpha-blocker and beta-blocker:*
   a. Labetalol (Trandate, Normodyne)
   b. Carvedilol (Coreg)
5. *Neuronal-inhibiting drugs:*
   a. Guanadrel (Hylorel)
   b. Guanethidine (Ismelin)
   c. Reserpine (Serpasil)

Unfavorable Effects (Over 5:18 CHD Relative Risk Ratio)

1. *Diuretics (selected):*
   a. Chlorthalidone (Hygroton, Thalitone)
   b. Loop diuretics (furosemide, bumetanide, ethacrynic acid, torsemide)
   c. Quinazolines (metolazone)
   d. Thiazides (HCTZ, chlorothiazide, cyclothiazide, polythiazide, methyclothiazide)
2. *Beta-blockers without ISA:*
   a. Atenolol (Tenormin)
   b. Betaxolol (Kerlone)
   c. Metoprolol (Lopressor, Toprol XL)
   d. Nadolol (Corgard)
   e. Propranolol (Inderal, Inderal LA)
   f. Timolol (Blocadren)
   g. Bisoprolol (Zebeta)
3. *Beta-blockers with ISA:*
   a. Acebutolol (Sectral)
   b. Penbutolol (Levatol)
   c. Pindolol (Visken)
   d. Carteolol (Cartrol)

Calcium Channel Blockers and Atherosclerosis (Coronary Heart Disease Reduction)

Nifedipine vs. propranolol vs. isosorbide[85]	CHD/angina
Nifedipine vs. placebo (INTACT)[86]	Mild CHD/angina
Nifedipine vs. placebo (INTACT2)[125]	Mild CHD/angina
Verapamil vs. non–calcium channel blocker[87]	CHD/angina
Verapamil vs. placebo (FIPS)[87]	CHD/angina
Isradipine vs. HCTZ (MIDAS)[88]	Carotid artery
Nicardipine vs. placebo[89]	CHD
Verapamil vs. chlorthalidone (VHAS)	CHD/CVD/carotid
Amlodipine vs. Placebo (PREVENT)	CHD/CVD/carotid

CCB reduce CHD obstruction and carotid artery obstruction compared to placebo-treated or diuretic-treated hypertensive patients as assessed with arteriography or ultrasound.

Hypertension and Renal Damage[4,5,90–93,118,119,137-146]

1. Hypertensive arteriolar nephrosclerosis accounts for 25% to 30% of all end-stage renal disease in the United States (more prevalent in African-Americans than in whites).[137,139]

2. No data show a reduction in end-stage renal disease related to the treatment of stage I-II mild to moderate hypertension.

3. Clinical trials,[5] both prospective and retrospective, suggest that 15% to 35% of patients with mild to moderate hypertension progress to renal insufficiency on stepped-care therapy (diuretics and beta-blockers) despite adequate BP control. This is particularly true for African-American hypertensive patients.

4. It has been suggested that chronic elevations of intraglomerular capillary pressure (IGCP) lead to loss of glomeruli and nephron function. The relative resistance of the afferent (preglomerular) and efferent (postglomerular) arteriole determines the IGCP.

5. As BP increases, there is a progressive rise in RVR, decreases in effective RBF and renal plasma flow (RPF), and a later decrease in GFR. Once renal mass losses exceed 50%, autoregulation is impaired, and preglomerular capillary vasodilation induces structural and functional hypertrophy of residual intact nephrons. Hyperperfusion, hyperfiltration, and elevated IGCP ensue, mediating glomerular injury.

6. Antihypertensive therapy that normalizes BP and preserves the autoregulatory ability of the preglomerular arteriole and the normal relation of afferent to efferent resistance should provide renal protection.

7. Angiotensin II and catecholamines regulate efferent arteriolar constriction. Drugs that interfere with angiotensin II or

catecholamine actions (ACE inhibitors, Ang-II inhibitors, and calcium channel blockers) may offer some renal protection, whereas drugs that increase angiotensin II or catecholamine levels (diuretics) may induce renal damage. Drugs that cause regression of glomerular and renal vascular hypertrophy may improve renal function (ARBs, ACE inhibitors, and calcium channel blockers).

8. Studies have shown that calcium channel blockers with ARB or ACE inhibitor therapy in hypertensive patients prevent the decline in GFR with time better than beta-blockers and diuretics.[90,118,119] CCB, ACEI and ARB monotherapy are also better than diuretics or beta-blockers. This is also true in patients with chronic renal disease, with proteinuria, with diabetes, and in hypertensive diabetics.[131,132]

9. Both SBP and DBP correlate with the development and progression of renal insufficiency and failure, but SBP is more important than DBP as a risk factor.[138] Any degree of hypertension may cause renal impairment.

10. The progression of hypertensive nephrosclerosis is reduced proportionately to the reduction in blood pressure. Target BP should be 110-120/70-75 mm Hg in hypertensive patients with renal impairment and in hypertensive diabetics. [140-146]

Hypertension-Related Renal Damage: Postulated Mechanisms[4,5,90–93]

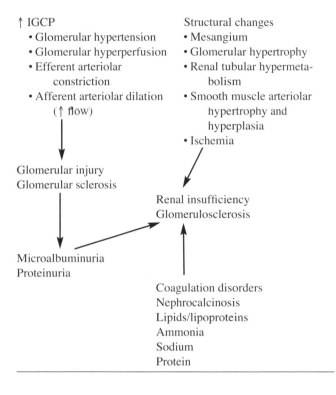

↑ IGCP
- Glomerular hypertension
- Glomerular hyperperfusion
- Efferent arteriolar constriction
- Afferent arteriolar dilation (↑ flow)

Structural changes
- Mesangium
- Glomerular hypertrophy
- Renal tubular hypermetabolism
- Smooth muscle arteriolar hypertrophy and hyperplasia
- Ischemia

Glomerular injury
Glomerular sclerosis

Renal insufficiency
Glomerulosclerosis

Microalbuminuria
Proteinuria

Coagulation disorders
Nephrocalcinosis
Lipids/lipoproteins
Ammonia
Sodium
Protein

Hypertension, Renal Disease, and Antihypertensive Therapy

Study	Result
Diuretics and beta-blockers[90]	16% with normal BP developed progressive renal insufficiency.
Diuretic vs. calcium channel blocker, minoxidil[91]	Faster rate of decline of renal function on diuretics. Calcium channel blocker or minoxidil: 40% slower rate of decline in renal function.
Calcium channel blocker (nisoldipine)[92]	Calcium channel blocker slowed or improved renal function compared to beta-blocker, alpha-blocker, hydralazine.
Calcium channel blocker, clonidine, minoxidil vs. beta-blocker, alpha-blocker, diuretic[91]	Calcium channel blocker, clonidine, minoxidil slowed renal function decline when added to diuretic. Beta-blockers or alpha-blocker did not.
Diuretic with or without beta-blocker[93]	Proteinuria and renal insufficiency despite BP control.
Calcium channel bocker with ACE I[124,131,132]	Provides additional renal protection above monotherapy
CCB, ACEI and ARB studies (various)[140-146]	

Effects of Antihypertensive Drugs on Renal Function[4,5]

	Diuretics	Beta-Blockers	Beta-Blockers with ISA	Beta-Blockers + Alpha Blockers	Direct Vasodilators	Neuronal Inhibitors	Calcium Channel Blockers	A-II Inhibitors + ACE Inhibitors	Central Alpha-Agonists	Alpha Methyldopa	Alpha-Blockers
GFR	→	→/↓	↑	↑	→/↑	↓	↓	→	↑/→	↑/→	→/↑
ERPF	→	→/↓	↑	↑	→/↑	→	←	←	↑	↑	→/↑
GFR/ERPF	↑	↑	↑	↑	↑	→	↑	↑	↑	↑	↑
RBF	→	→/↓	→/↑	→/↑	→/↑	→	?/→	↓/→	↑/→	↑/→	→/?
RVR	←	→/↑	↑	↑	→	→	↓/↑	→	→/↑	→	↑
IGCP	←	?	?	?	←	?	↓/↑	→	?	?	?
Urinary albumin	←	?	?	?	←	?	→/↑	←	?	?	?
Urinary$_{Na}^{+}$	←	→/↑	→/↓	↑	↑	→/↓	←	→	→/↑	→	↑/↓
Urinary$_{K}^{+}$	←	→/↓	↑	↑	↑	↑	→/↑	→	↑	↑	↑
Urinary$_{Mg}^{2+}$	←	→/↓	↑	↑	↑	↑	↑	→	↑	↑	↑
Plasma volume	←	→/↑	→/↑	→/↑	↑	→/↓	→	→/↓	→/↓	←	↑

ERPF, Effective renal plasma flow.
↓ Reduced; ↑ increased; → no change; ? unknown.

53

Hypertension and Diabetes Mellitus

Causes of Death Among People with Diabetes

Cause	% of Deaths
Ischemic heart disease	40
Other heart disease	15
Diabetes (acute complications)	13
Cancer	13
Cerebrovascular disease	10
Pneumonia/influenza	4
All other causes	5

From Geiss LS, et al: Mortality in non-insulin-dependent diabetes. Diabetes in America, 2nd ed. Bethesda, MD, National Diabetes Data Group, 1995, pp 233–257. The book is also available online.

Major CV Events in Patients with Diabetes in Relation to Target Blood Pressure Groups

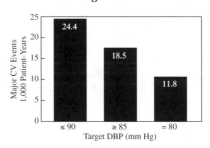

JNC VI Recommendations for Patients with Diabetes Mellitus

- Reduce BP < 130/85 mm Hg
  Lifestyle modification (especially weight loss)
  ACEIs, beta-blockers, calcium antagonists, and low-dose diuretics preferred

- In patients with diabetic nephropathy ACEIs preferred

Large Clinical Trials in Hypertension and Type 2 Diabetes or Impaired Glucose Metabolism

HOT	SYST-EUR
UKPDS	SHEP
CAPPP	

HOT — Rate of Major CV Events According to Randomized Groups

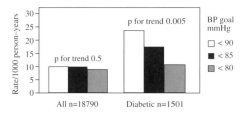

From Hansson L, Zanchetti A, Carruthers SG, et al. Effects of intensive blood-pressure lowering and low-dose aspirin in patients with hypertension: Principal results of the Hypertension Optimal Treatment (HOT) randomised trial. Lancet. 1998;351:1755–1762, with permission.

UK Prospective Diabetes Study

Tight vs less tight BP control

Endpoint	RR	95% CI
Any endpoint	0.76	0.62–0.92
Diabetes death	0.68	0.49–0.94
Any death	0.82	0.63–1.08
MI	0.79	0.59–1.07
Stroke	0.56	0.35–0.89
PAD	0.51	0.19–1.37
Microvascular disease	0.63	0.44–0.89

n = 758 vs 390.

From UK Prospective Diabetes Study Group. Tight blood pressure control and risk of macrovascular and microvascular complications in type 2 diabetes: UKPDS 38. BMJ. 1998;317:703–713, with permission.

UK Prospective Diabetes Study

| | Captopril vs Atenolol | |
Endpoint	RR	95% CI
Any endpoint	1.10	0.86–1.41
Diabetes death	1.27	0.82–1.97
Any death	1.14	0.81–1.61
MI	1.20	0.82–1.76
Stroke	1.12	0.59–2.12
PAD	1.48	0.35–6.19
Microvascular disease	1.29	0.80–2.10

n = 400 vs 358.

From UK Prospective Diabetes Study Group. Efficacy of atenolol and captopril in reducing risk of macrovascular and microvascular complications in type 2 diabetes: UKPDS 39. BMJ. 1998;317:713–720, with permission.

SYST-EUR
Systolic Hypertension in Europe Trial:
Effect of active treatment in diabetic (n=492)
and nondiabetic (n=4203) hypertensive patients (n=4695)
Median follow-up was 2 years

CCB treatment reduced stroke 69% and cardiac events
57% in diabetic hypertensives

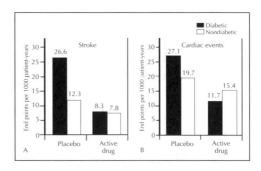

Benefit of active treatment began soon after randomization, when
most patients were still on monotherapy with nitrendipine.

Prisant LM, Louard RJ: Controversies surrounding the treatment of the hypertensive patient with diabetes. Current Hypertension Reports 1999, 1:512-520, with permission.

CAPPP — Patients with Diabetes[133*]

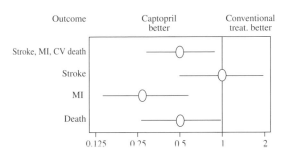

*See also charts on page 32.

SHEP

Systolic Hypertension in the Elderly Program:
Relative risk reduction of end points by active treatment versus placebo for diabetic (n=583) and nondiabetic (n=4149) patients by treatment group
Mean follow-up was 4.5 years

Diuretic with beta blocker treatment reduced cardiac events
54% but did *not* alter CVA morbidity
or mortality compared to placebo.

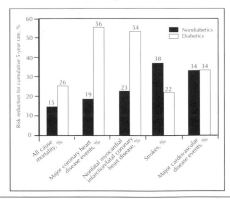

Prisant LM, Louard RJ: Controversies surrounding the treatment of the hypertensive patient with diabetes. Current Hypertension Reports 1999, 1:512-520, with permission.

Hypertensive Diabetics: Mortality and CHD and Antihypertensive Therapy[94]

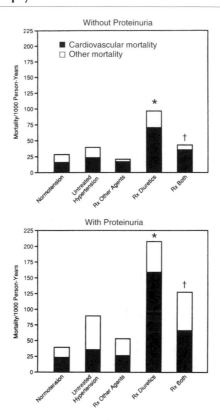

Mortality per 1000 person-years in diabetic patients without proteinuria and with proteinuria according to hypertension status and type of antihypertensive treatment (Rx) during each year of follow-up. Diuretics increased cardiovascular mortality and total mortality compared to other antihypertensive drugs or no treatment. *P < 0.025; †P<0.025 vs. treatment with diuretics alone. (From Warram JH, Laffel LMB, Valsania P, et al. Excess mortality associated with diuretic therapy in diabetes mellitus. Arch Intern Med 1991; 151:1350–1356, with permission.)

Selection of Therapy Based on Subsets of Hypertension

Selection of antihypertensive therapy based on the subsets of hypertension approach allows for the categorization of drugs into three groups: drugs of choice, alternatives, and contraindicated drugs. Diseases in the left-hand column are often associated with hypertension. A drug should be selected considering all disease factors. Drugs are listed in *alphabetical order*, not by preference, in each column.

Concomitant Condition	Drug(s) of Choice	Alternatives	Relative or Absolute Contraindication
Addictive Syndromes: withdrawal from tobacco, alcohol, opiates	Central alpha-agonist (clonidine)		
Angina: mixed	Beta-blocker without ISA Calcium channel blocker	Ang-II blocker ACE inhibitor Alpha-blocker Central alpha-agonist Diuretic Alpha- and beta-blocker	Beta-blocker with ISA Direct vasodilators Neuronal inhibitors Reserpine
Angina: obstructive	Beta-blocker without ISA Calcium channel blocker	Ang-II blocker ACE inhibitor Alpha-blocker Central alpha-agonist Diuretic Alpha- and beta-blocker	Beta-blocker with ISA Direct vasodilators Neuronal inhibitors Reserpine
Angina: vasospastic	Calcium channel blocker	Ang-II blocker ACE inhibitor Alpha-blocker Central alpha-agonist Diuretic	Beta-blocker without ISA Beta-blocker with ISA Direct vasodilator Alpha- and beta-blocker Neuronal inhibitor Reserpine

Concomitant Condition	Drug(s) of Choice	Alternatives	Relative or Absolute Contraindication
Anxiety/Stress	Central alpha-agonist Beta-blocker without ISA		
Supraventricular tachycardia	Central alpha-agonist Nondihydropyridine calcium channel blocker	ACE inhibitor Alpha-blocker Amlodipine Diuretic Felodipine Alpha- and beta-blocker Nicardipine Nifedipine Nisoldipine Reserpine	Direct vasodilator Neuronal inhibitor
Cerebrovascular disease	ACE inhibitor Calcium channel blocker Ang-II blocker	Alpha-blocker Central alpha-agonist Direct vasodilator Alpha- and beta-blocker	Beta-blocker without ISA Beta-blocker with ISA Diuretic Neuronal inhibitor Reserpine
Chronic liver disease	Alpha-blocker Calcium channel blocker Central alpha-agonist	ACE inhibitor Direct vasodilator Diuretic Alpha- and beta-blocker	Beta-blocker Methyldopa Neuronal inhibitor Reserpine
CHF (systolic failure)	Ang-II blocker ACE inhibitor Amlodipine Carvedilol Direct vasodilator Diuretic Spironolactone	Alpha-blocker Central alpha-agonist Calcium channel blocker Isradipine Nicardipine Nifedipine Nisoldipine Beta-blocker without ISA	Beta-blocker with ISA Alpha- and beta-blocker Neuronal inhibitor Reserpine Verapamil Diltiazem
Cyclosporine-induced hypertension	Calcium channel blocker		

Concomitant Condition	Drug(s) of Choice	Alternatives	Relative or Absolute Contraindication
Depression	Ang-II blocker ACE inhibitor Alpha-blocker Calcium channel blocker	Central alpha-agonist Diuretic Direct vaso-dilator	Beta-blocker without ISA Beta-blocker with ISA Alpha- and beta-blocker Methyldopa Neuronal inhibitor Reserpine
Diabetes mellitus	Ang-II blocker? ACE inhibitor Alpha-blocker Calcium channel blocker Central alpha-agonist	Beta-blocker with ISA Direct vasodilator Indapamide Alpha- and beta-blocker	Beta-blocker without ISA Diuretic Methyldopa Neuronal inhibitor Reserpine
Diabetic diarrhea and gustatory sweating	Central alpha-agonist (clonidine)		
Diastolic dysfunction or failure	Calcium channel blocker	Ang-II blocker ACE inhibitor Alpha-blocker Beta-blocker without ISA Central alpha-agonist Alpha- and beta-blocker	Beta-blocker with ISA Direct vasodilator Diuretic Neuronal inhibitor Reserpine
Dyslipidemia	Alpha-blocker Calcium channel blocker Central alpha-agonist	Ang-II blocker ACE inhibitor Beta-blocker with ISA Alpha- and beta-blocker Direct vasodilator Indapamide	Beta-blocker without ISA Diuretic Methyldopa Neuronal inhibitor Reserpine

Concomitant Condition	Drug(s) of Choice	Alternatives	Relative or Absolute Contraindication
Essential tremor	Central alpha-agonist Beta-blocker without ISA		
Glaucoma	Beta-blocker Central alpha-agonist Diuretic		
Hyperuricemia	Ang-II blocker ACE inhibitor Alpha-blocker Calcium channel blocker Central alpha agonist	Direct vaso-dilator Alpha- and beta-blocker Neuronal inhibitor Reserpine	Beta-blocker without ISA Beta-blocker with ISA Diuretic
Hyper-thyroidism	Beta-blocker		
Exercise	Ang-II blocker ACE inhibitor Alpha-blocker Calcium channel blocker Central alpha-agonist	Beta-blocker with ISA Diuretic Direct vaso-dilator Alpha- and beta-blocker Methyldopa	Beta-blocker without ISA Neuronal inhibitor Reserpine
LVH	Ang-II blocker ACE inhibitor Alpha-blocker Calcium channel blocker Central alpha-agonist Indapamide Alpha- and beta-blocker	Beta-blocker without ISA Reserpine Diuretic	Beta-blocker with ISA Direct vaso-dilator Neuronal inhibitor

Concomitant Condition	Drug(s) of Choice	Alternatives	Relative or Absolute Contraindication
Menopausal symptoms	Central alpha-agonist (clonidine)		Direct vasodilator
Microvascular angina	Calcium channel blocker	Ang-II blocker ACE inhibitor Alpha-blocker Central alpha-agonist	Beta-blocker without ISA Beta-blocker with ISA Direct vaso-dilator Diuretic Alpha- and beta-blocker Neuronal inhibitor Reserpine
Migraine headache (prophylaxis)	Beta-blocker without ISA Calcium channel blocker Central alpha-agonist	Ang-II blocker ACE inhibitor Alpha-blocker Beta-blocker with ISA Diuretic Alpha-and beta-blocker	Direct vaso-dilator Neuronal inhibitor Reserpine
Mitral valve prolapse	Beta-blocker without ISA Calcium channel blocker Central alpha-agonist	Ang-II blocker ACE inhibitor Alpha-blocker Alpha- and beta-blocker	Beta-blocker with ISA Direct vaso-dilator Diuretic Neuronal inhibitor Reserpine
Obesity	ACE inhibitor Ang-II blocker Alpha-blocker Calcium channel blocker Central alpha-agonist	Direct vaso-dilator Diuretic Alpha- and beta-blocker	Beta-blocker without ISA Beta-blocker with ISA Neuronal inhibitor Reserpine

Concomitant Condition	Drug(s) of Choice	Alternatives	Relative or Absolute Contraindication
Obstructive airway disease	Alpha-blocker Calcium channel blocker Central alpha-agonist	Ang-II blocker ACE inhibitor Direct vaso-dilator Diuretic	Beta-blocker without ISA Beta-blocker with ISA Alpha- and beta-blocker Neuronal inhibitor Reserpine
Peptic ulcer disease	Calcium channel blocker Central alpha-agonist	Ang-II blocker ACE inhibitor Alpha-blocker Beta-blocker Direct vaso-dilator Diuretic Alpha- and beta-blocker	Neuronal inhibitor Reserpine
Peripheral vascular disease	Calcium channel blocker	Ang-II blocker ACE inhibitor Alpha-blocker Central alpha-agonist Direct vaso-dilator Diuretic	Beta-blocker without ISA Beta-blocker with ISA Alpha- and beta-blocker Neuronal inhibitor Reserpine
Post-MI: non–Q-wave Normal left-ventricular function	Diltiazem? Verapamil? ACE inhibitor Ang-II antagonist?	Alpha-blocker Beta-blocker without ISA Central alpha-agonist Calcium channel blocker Amlodipine Isradipine Nicardipine Nifedipine Nisoldipine Alpha- and beta-blocker	Beta-blocker with ISA Direct vaso-dilator Diuretic Neuronal inhibitor Reserpine

Concomitant Condition	Drug(s) of Choice	Alternatives	Relative or Absolute Contraindication
Abnormal left ventricular function	Ang-II blocker Ace inhibitor Diuretic		
Post-MI: Q-wave Normal left ventricular function	ACEI ARB Beta-blocker without ISA	Calcium channel blocker Central alpha-agonist Alpha- and beta-blocker	Beta-blocker with ISA Direct vaso-dilator Diuretic Neuronal inhibitor Reserpine
Abnormal left ventricular function	Ang-II blocker ACE inhibitor Diuretic		
Pregnancy (first and second trimester)	Hydralazine Methyldopa Central alpha-agonist	Possibly alpha-blocker, calcium channel blocker*	Ang-II antagonist ACE inhibitor Beta-blocker without ISA Beta-blocker with ISA Diuretic Alpha- and beta-blocker Neuronal inhibitor Reserpine
Premature ventricular contractions	Beta-blocker without ISA Calcium channel blocker Verapamil	Ang-II blocker ACE inhibitor Alpha-blocker Central alpha-agonist Alpha- and beta-blocker Diltiazem Nifedipine	Beta-blocker with ISA Direct vaso-dilator Diuretic Neuronal inhibitor Reserpine
Prostatism	Alpha-blocker		
Proteinuria	ACE inhibitor Ang-II blocker	Verapamil Amlodipine	Diuretic Beta-blocker

Concomitant Condition	Drug(s) of Choice	Alternatives	Relative or Absolute Contraindication
Pulmonary hypertension	Dihydropyridine Calcium channel blockers Amlodipine Nifedipine Direct vaso-dilator	Ang-II blocker ACE inhibitor Alpha-blocker Central alpha-agonist Diuretic Alpha- and beta-blocker	Beta-blocker
Raynaud's phenomenon	DHP-Calcium channel blockers Amlodidine Nifedipine	Ang-II blocker ACE inhibitor Alpha-blocker Central alpha-agonist Direct vaso-dilator Neuronal inhibitor Reserpine	Beta-blocker without ISA Beta-blocker with ISA Alpha- and beta-blocker
Renal insufficiency	ACE inhibitor Alpha-blocker Ang-II antagonist Calcium channel blocker Central alpha-agonist	Direct vaso-dilator Diuretic[†] Alpha- and beta-blocker	Beta-blocker without ISA Beta-blocker with ISA Neuronal inhibitor Reserpine
Renovascular disease (renal artery disease)	Calcium channel blocker Central alpha-agonist Alpha blocker	Beta-blocker Diuretic	ACE inhibitor Ang-II blocker
Sexual dysfunction	Ang-II antagonist ACE inhibitor Alpha-blocker Calcium channel blocker	Central alpha-agonist Direct vaso-dilator Diuretic	Beta-blocker without ISA Beta-blocker with ISA Alpha- and beta-blocker Methyldopa Neuronal inhibitor Reserpine

Concomitant Condition	Drug(s) of Choice	Alternatives	Relative or Absolute Contraindication
Sick sinus syndrome or atrio-ventricular (AV) block	Ang-II blocker ACE inhibitor Alpha-blocker Amlodipine Isradipine Nicardipine Nisoldipine	Calcium channel blocker Direct vaso-dilator Diuretic	Beta-blocker without ISA Beta-blocker with ISA Central alpha-agonist Calcium channel blocker Diltiazem Verapamil Alpha- and beta-blocker Neuronal inhibitor Reserpine
Sinusitis/rhinitis	Central alpha-agonist	Ang-II blocker ACE inhibitor Alpha-blocker Calcium channel blocker Direct vaso-dilator Diuretic	Beta-blocker Alpha- and beta-blocker Neuronal inhibitor Reserpine
Toxemia of pregnancy (eclampsia)	Central alpha-agonist Calcium channel blocker* Hydralazine Methyldopa	Alpha-blocker*	ACE inhibitor Beta-blocker without ISA Beta-blocker with ISA Diuretic Alpha- and beta-blocker Neuronal inhibitor Reserpine
GERD	ACEI ARB	Alpha-blocker Diuretic Beta-blocker Central alpha-agonist	CCB (decreased LES tone)

Concomitant Condition	Drug(s) of Choice	Alternatives	Relative or Absolute Contraindication
Use of NSAIDs	Calcium channel blocker	Alpha-blocker Central alpha-agonist	Ang-II antagonists ACE inhibitor Beta-blocker with ISA Beta-blocker without ISA Direct vaso-dilator Diuretic Alpha- and beta-blocker Neuronal inhibitor Reserpine
Volume overload	Ang-II blocker ACE inhibitor Calcium channel blocker Diuretic	Alpha-blocker Central alpha-agonist Alpha- and beta-blocker	Beta-blocker Direct vaso-dilator Neuronal inhibitor Reserpine

*These products are not approved for use during pregnancy.
†Use caution in renal artery stenosis (bilateral) and severe chronic renal impairment; monitor K^+ levels.

Demographics and Antihypertensive Drugs

Demographic Profile	Drug(s) of Choice	Alternatives	Relative or Absolute Contra-indication
*Young patient	Ang-II blocker ACE inhibitor Alpha-blocker Calcium channel blocker Central alpha agonist	Beta-blocker with ISA Direct vaso-dilator Alpha- and beta-blocker	Beta-blocker without ISA Diuretic Neuronal inhibitor Reserpine
Elderly patient	Alpha-blocker Calcium channel blocker Central alpha-agonist	Ang-II blocker ACE blocker Beta-blocker without ISA Beta-blocker with ISA Diuretic Alpha- and beta-blocker	Direct vaso-dilator Neuronal inhibitor Reserpine
African-American patient	Alpha-blocker Calcium channel blocker Central alpha-agonist	Ang-II blocker ACE blocker Direct vaso-dilator	Beta-blocker with ISA Beta-blocker without ISA Alpha- and beta-blocker Neuronal inhibitor Reserpine
White patient	Ang-II blocker ACE blocker Alpha-blocker Calcium channel blocker Central alpha-agonist	Direct vaso-dilator Alpha- and beta-blocker Diuretic	Beta-blocker with ISA Beta-blocker without ISA Neuronal inhibitor Reserpine

*Unless pregnant, then avoid ACEI, ARB, BB, and diuretic.

Resistant Hypertension

Definition

The patient's DBP remains above 90 mm Hg despite full doses of three appropriate antihypertensive medications and has been documented on at least two separate visits in the office under proper conditions *and* out of the office with home BP monitoring or 24-hour ambulatory blood pressure monitoring (ABPM).

Causes

An inadequate drug regimen and patient noncompliance account for 70% of total causes.

1. Patient noncompliance to therapy
2. Inadequate drug regimen
   a. Drug doses too low
   b. Drug interactions—antihypertensive agents (Two central alpha-agonists, two ACE I or beta-blockers and central alpha-agonist with beta-blocker)
   c. Rapid metabolism or inactivation (hydralazine)
   d. Other drug interactions and interfering agents
      (1) Corticosteroids and anabolic steroids
      (2) Aldosterone (florinef)
      (3) Sympathomimetics and phenylpropanolamine
      (4) NSAIDs (ACE I, beta-blockers, diuretics)
      (5) Antidepressants—tricyclics and central alpha-agonist
      (6) Decongestants—pseudoephedrine, nasal sprays
      (7) Excess alcohol ingestion (over 30 mL/day) for 7-10 weeks
      (8) Excess caffeine ingestion (variable)
      (9) Excess tobacco use (variable)
      (10) Oral contraceptives
      (11) Erythropoietin
      (12) Cyclosporine
      (13) MAO inhibitors and phenothiazines
      (14) Cocaine and amphetamines
      (15) Appetite suppressants
      (16) Omeprazole (Prilosec)

3. Volume overload states
   a. Inadequate diuretic therapy
   b. High sodium intake (10 to 15 g/day)
   c. Secondary to BP reduction with some agents (direct vasodilators) and some beta-blockers pseudotolerance caused by reflex volume overload, tachycardia, or vasoconstriction)
   d. Nephrosclerosis and CRF

4. Obesity and rapid weight gain

5. Secondary hypertension (10%)
   a. Renovascular hypertension (most common)
   b. Renal insufficiency and failure
   c. Pheochromocytoma
   d. Primary aldosteronism
   e. Cushing's syndrome
   f. Coarctation of aorta
   g. Sleep apnea
   h. Thyroid disease
   i. Hypercalcemia
   j. Licorice intoxication (in chewing tobacco)

6. Pseudo resistance
   a. Using regular adult cuff on obese arm
   b. White coat hypertension
   c. Pseudohypertension in elderly

7. Miscellaneous
   a. Chronic anxiety, panic attacks
   b. Chronic pain
   c. Diffuse vasoconstriction (arteritis)
   d. Insulin resistance
   e. Inappropriate diuretic in patients with renal insufficiency and creatinine clearance below 30 cc/min (i.e., thiazine)

Hypertensive Urgencies and Emergencies

Definitions

1. *Hypertensive urgency:* DBP ≥120 mm Hg in the absence of significant end-organ damage.
   a. Grade I or II Keith-Wagener fundoscopic changes
   b. Postoperative hypertension
   c. Preoperative hypertension
   d. Pain-induced or stress-induced hypertension
2. *Hypertensive emergency:* DBP >120 mm Hg with one of following:
   a. Intracranial hemorrhage or thrombotic CVA
   b. Subarachnoid bleed
   c. Hypertensive encephalopathy
   d. Acute aortic dissection
   e. Acute pulmonary edema, acute CHF, and acute left ventricular failure
   f. Eclampsia (toxemia of pregnancy)
   g. Pheochromocytoma hypertensive crisis
   h. Grade III or IV Keith-Wagener fundoscopic changes
   i. Acute renal insufficiency or failure
   j. Myocardial insufficiency syndromes (unstable angina pectoris, acute MI)
   k. Hematuria

Precipitating Factors in Hypertensive Crisis

1. Accelerated sudden rise in blood pressure in a patient with preexisting essential hypertension
2. Renovascular hypertension
3. Glomerulonephritis—acute
4. Eclampsia
5. Pheochromocytoma
6. Antihypertensive withdrawal syndromes

7. Head injuries
8. Renin secreting tumors
9. Ingestion of catecholamine precursors in patients taking MAO inhibitors

Malignant Hypertension

1. Fundoscopic changes of necrotizing arteriolitis (hemorrhages, exudates), disc edema, and papilledema (visual changes, nausea, vomiting, headache, confusion, somnolence, stupor, neurologic deficits, seizures, coma).
2. Hypertensive encephalopathy
3. Diastolic blood pressure > 120 mm Hg with target organ damage
4. Decreasing renal function, proteinuria, hematuria, casts, oliguria, azotemia
5. Microangiopathic hemolytic anemia
6. Left ventricular failure and CHF and pulmonary edema

Factors That Constitute Malignant Hypertension

1. Absolute level of blood pressure
2. Rate of development of blood pressure
3. Type and level of vasoactive substances
4. Presence of end-organ damage

Pathophysiology

High blood pressure level

+

Increased vascular reactivity

+

Critical circulating levels of vasoactive and "vasculotoxic" agents (angiotensin II, NE, vasopressin)

↓

Relative narrowing efferent arteriole

↓

Sodium "pressure" diuresis (differential effect on afferent and efferent renal arteriole)

↓

Hypovolemia

↓

Increased angiotensin II ± norepinephrine ± vasopressin

Narrowing in interlobular arteries

↑

Proliferation of myointimal cells

↑

Migration of myointimal cells to lumen

↑

Platelet and fibrin migration and mitogenic factors

↑

Platelet and fibrin deposition

"Sausage-string" change in arteries

↓

Endothelial damage and platelet aggregation

↓

Release of platelet factors and thromboxane

↓

Microangiopathic hemolytic anemia and intravascular coagulation

Treatment: General Principles

Balance the benefit of immediate reduction in BP to prevent irreversible organ damage against the risk of marked decrease in perfusion and blood flow to vital organs, particularly to the brain, myocardium, and kidney or regional blood flow changes within each organ.

1. Reduce DBP to no less than 100 mm Hg, the SBP to no less than 160 mm Hg, or the MAP to no less than 120 mm Hg the first 24 to 48 hours except in hypertensive emergencies as indicated. Attempt an average reduction of 25% below baseline BP or to the minimum BP indicated above.

2. Acute lowering of blood pressure may decrease blood flow to the brain, myocardium, and kidneys.

3. Attempt to establish normotension within a few days.

4. Avoid hypotension or normotension during first 24 hours except in hypertensive emergencies as indicated.

5. Parenteral or oral antihypertensives are appropriate depending on the clinical setting.

6. Begin concomitant long-term therapy soon after the initial emergency treatment.

7. Assess volume status of patient. Do not overuse diuretics, and avoid sodium restriction in the early phases of malignant hypertension.

8. Reflex volume retention may occur after a few days on some nondiuretic antihypertensive drugs, such as beta-blockers and direct vasodilators—concept of pseudotolerance.

Treatment: Rapidity of Onset

1. Aortic dissection.

2. Pulmonary edema (caution in acute MI).

3. Malignant hypertension in certain clinical settings with encephalopathy, papilledema—controlled reduction.

4. Subarachnoid bleed or intracerebral bleed—controversial.

Treatment: Choice of Drug

1. Rapidity of blood pressure drop desired and level of blood pressure.
2. Duration of action of antihypertensive agent.
3. Hemodynamic effect of drug (i.e., use in presence of pulmonary edema, CHF, angina, MI, CVA, aortic dissection, renal insufficiency).
4. Effect on RBF, GRF, and function.
5. Potential and known adverse effects.

Acute Nonparenteral Therapy

Drugs	Route	Onset	Maximum Effect	Duration	Dosage
Clonidine (Catapres)	Oral	30 min	1–2 hr	8–12 hr	0.1–0.2 mg initial then 0.05–0.1 mg q hr to maximum 0.8 mg
Nitroglycerin (Nitrostat)	Sublingual	1 min	15 min	1 hr	$\frac{1}{150}$ grain

*Use with caution, if at all.

Acute Parenteral Therapy

Drugs	Route	Onset	Maximum Effect	Duration	Dosage
*Sodium nitroprusside (Nipride, Nitropress)	IV	seconds	1–2 min	3–5 min	16 µg/min to 1–6 µg/kg/min
*Fenoldopam mesylate (Corlopam)	IV	< 5 min	5–10 min	30 min	0.1–0.3 µg/kg per min
Trimethaphan (Arfonad)	IV	1–5 min	2–5 min	10 min	0.5–5 mg/min
Diazoxide (Hyperstat)	IV	1–5 min	2–3 min	4–24 hr	50 mg IV q 5–10 min
			Bolus infusion		7.5–30 mg/min + propranolol load
			Infusion method		
Hydralazine (Apresoline)	IV	10–20 min	20–40 min	3–8 hr	10 to 20 mg
Methyldopa (Aldomet)	IV	2–3 hr	3–5 hr	6–12 hr	250–500 mg q 6 hr
Phentolamine (Regitine)	IV	(for catecholamine excess)			load 5–10 mg IV q 5 min, infuse 0.2–0.5 mg/min
Labetalol (Trandate, Normodyne)	IV	5 min	5–10 min	3–6 hr	2 mg/min IV infusion or 20 mg q 10 min to a maximum 80 mg q 10 min Maximum cumulative dose 300 mg may not be effective in severely hypertensive patients already receiving other antihypertensive agents (propranolol, prazosin)
Nicardipine (Cardene)	IV	10 min	30 min	3–6 hr	5 mg/hr increased 1–2.5 mg/hr every 15 min up to 15 mg/hr
Nitroglycerin	IV	1–2 min	—	2–3 min	5–100 µg/min
Dilevalol	IV	1–5 min	—	3–6 hr	10 mg followed by 25–100 mg every 15 min
Enalapril AT	IV	10 min	1–4 hr	2–6 hr	1.25 mg then 2.5 to 10 mg every 30–60 min
Esmolol hydrochloride	IV	1–2 min	5 min	10–20 min	250–500 µg/kg/min for 1 min then 50–100 µg/kg/min for 4 min; may repeat sequence

77

*Preferred drugs

Treatment of Specific Hypertensive Disorders

1.	Hypertension + Congestive heart failure	Nitroglycerin IV Sodium nitroprusside and loop diuretics DHP-CCB, amlodipine Clonidine ACEI ARB
2.	Hypertension + Coronary insufficiency	Non DHP-CCB Nitroglycerin Beta-blockers Clonidine
3.	Aortic dissection aneurysm	Trimethaphan + propranolol or Nitroprusside + propranolol Labetalol or esmolol
4.	Catecholamine excess (pheochromocytoma)	Phentolamine
5.	Hypertension alone	Fenoldopam Sodium nitroprusside Labetalol-parenteral alternate Nicardipine Nitroglycerin Clonidine (urgency)

Hypertension in Pregnancy

Classification

1. Pregnancy–induced hypertension (PIH) or gestational hypertension.
2. Chronic hypertension: Preexisting, before 20 weeks' gestation.
3. Preeclampsia: Hypertension with proteinuria and edema. Occurs after 20th week of gestation (usually after 36th week).
4. Eclampsia: Preeclampsia + convulsions, coma

Definition

1. BP usually falls during the first and second trimester.
2. PIH occurs if BP rises more than 30/15 mm Hg or MAP >25 mm Hg or to a level above 140/90 in the last trimester.
3. Most PIH occurs after the 35th week.
4. Preeclampsia develops after 20th week.
5. About 10% of pregnancies are complicated by hypertension.

Pathogenesis: Preeclampsia

1. Increased sensitivity to pressure effects of angiotensin II
2. Reduced intravascular volume
3. Decreased PRA
4. Decreased prostacyclin/thromboxane ratio
5. Increased atrial natriuretic peptide
6. Increased endothelin
7. Decreased endothelin relaxing factor (nitrous oxide)
8. Activation of coagulation
9. Increased fibrin degradation products
10. Thrombocytopenia
11. Increased factor XII
12. Decreased factor X and XI
13. Increased fibrinogen
14. High fibronectin
15. Low antithrombin III
16. Low alpha, antiplasmin
17. Increased plasminogen activator inhibitor activity
18. Vasospasm
19. Reduced cardiac output
20. Increased peripheral vascular resistance
21. Decreased sodium exchange
22. Decreased renal blood flow
23. Decreased glomerular filtration
24. Hyperuricemia

Generalized reduced organ perfusion occurs with widespread hemorrhage and necrosis in brain, liver, heart, and kidney with vascular endothelial damage and marked vasoconstriction of small arterioles. Preeclampsia may be a result of abnormal trophoblastic implantation and immunologic disorder.

Disease Spectrum: Preeclampsia

Clinical spectrum of coagulation disorders varies from thrombocytopenia to HELLP syndrome (hemolysis, elevated liver enzymes, low platelet count.)

Predisposing Factors

PIH

    a. Young primigravida   c. Diabetes mellitus
    b. Primary hypertension   d. Renal disease

Preeclampsia and eclampsia

    a. Extremes of reproductive age f. Chronic hypertension
    b. Nulliparas   g. Renal disease
    c. Multifetal pregnancy   h. Thalassemia and Rh
    d. Fetal hydrops   incompatibility
    e. Diabetes mellitus   i. Family history of preeclampsia

Management

1. PIH
   a. Do *not* restrict sodium.
   b. Bed rest and mild sedation, hospitalization.
   c. Avoid thiazide diuretics, beta-blockers, ACE inhibitors.
   d. Use hydralazine, methyldopa, clonidine, calcium channel blockers, alpha-blockers, ketanserin.

2. Preeclampsia and eclampsia
   a. Calcium supplement, 1–2 gm/day.
   b. Aspirin, 60–100 mg/day.
   c. Dipyridamole.
   d. Dipyridamole + heparin.
   e. Bed rest and sedation.
   f. Liberal sodium intake.
   g. $MgSO_4$ in eclampsia for convulsions and lower BP.
   h. Volume expansion: controversial (?).
   i. Medications to control BP: calcium channel blockers, clonidine, methyldopa, hydralazine, alpha-blockers (?).
   j. Avoid diuretics, beta-blockers, ACE inhibitors, and ARBs.

Quality of Life and Antihypertensive Therapy (Selected Trials)*

Study	Beta-Blocker	Diuretic	Central Alpha-Agonist	Calcium Channel Blocker	ACE[†] Inhibitor
MRC[39]	↓ (Propranolol)	→			
Croog[95]	↓ (Propranolol)	→	↓ (Methyldopa)		↑ (Captopril)
Jachuck[96]	↓ (Propranolol)	→	↓ (Methyldopa)		
Curb[97]		→	↓ (Methyldopa)		
Avorn[98]	↓ (Propranolol)				
Testa[99]	↓ (Atenolol)			↑ (Nifedipine)	
Os[100]				→ (Nifedipine)	→ (Lisinopril)
Croog[101]	→/↑ (Atenolol)			→/↑ (Verapamil)	→/↑ (Captopril)
Fletcher[102]	→ (Atenolol)				→ (Captopril)

*Quality of life is decreased with beta-blockers and diuretics but is unchanged or improved with ca cium channel blockers and ACE inhibitors.
†Quality of life with Ang-II receptor antagonists appears to be similar to ACE inhibitor.

Total Cost of Antihypertensive Therapy[5,117]

1. Acquisition cost.
2. Coprescription of secondary drugs.
3. Office visits.
4. Ancillary laboratory costs (electrolytes, glucose, lipids, ECG).
5. Costs to patient's lifestyle: quality of life and adverse effects.
6. Cost of increasing end-organ damage.
7. Mean costs per drug cost category—1-year use:[117]

	Acquisition Cost	Supplemental Drug Cost	Laboratory Cost	Clinic Visit Cost	Side Effect Cost	Total Cost
Diuretics	$133	$232	$117	$298	$263	$1043
β-Blockers	$334	$115	$56	$187	$203	$895
α-Blockers	$401	$290	$114	$227	$256	$1288
Centrally acting α-agonists	$285	$295	$125	$267	$193	$1165
ACE inhibitors + Ang-II receptor antagonists	$444	$291	$95	$218	$195	$1243
Calcium entry blockers	$540	$278	$87	$214	$306	$1425

Characteristics of the Ideal Antihypertensive Drug

1. Efficacious as monotherapy in more than 50% of all patients.
2. BP control during all activities for 24 hours.
3. Once-a-day dosing with high trough to peak ratio.
4. Hemodynamically logical and effective: Reduces SVR, improves arterial compliance, preserves CO, and maintains perfusion to all vital organs.
5. Lack of tolerance or pseudotolerance: No reflex volume retention or stimulation of neurohumoral mechanisms.
6. Favorable biochemical effects, metabolic effects, and risk factor profile.
7. Reverses structural, vascular smooth muscle, and cardiac hypertrophy; improves systolic and diastolic compliance and left ventricular contractility and function; reduces ventricular ectopy, if present.
8. Reduces all end-organ damage: cardiac, cerebrovascular, renal, retinal, and large artery.
9. Maintains normal hemodynamic response to aerobic and anaerobic exercise.
10. Low incidence of side effects, good quality of life.
11. Good compliance with drug regimen.
12. Good profile for concomitant diseases or problems.
13. Reasonable cost.
14. No withdrawal symptoms and prolongation of BP control with missed dose due to long biological half-life and efficacy of drug.

Combination Antihypertensive Therapy: Selected Drugs[125]

1. Calcium channel blocker plus:
   a. Alpha-blocker *or*
   b. ACE inhibitor, Ang-II receptor blocker or
   c. Central alpha-agonist
2. Alpha-blocker plus:
   a. Calcium channel blocker *or*
   b. ACE inhibitor, Ang-II receptor blocker
   c. Do not generally use with central alpha-agonist (reduced response rate)
3. Central alpha-agonist plus:
   a. Calcium channel blocker *or*
   b. ACE inhibitor, Ang-II receptor blocker
   c. Do not generally use with alpha-blocker (reduced response rate)
4. ACE inhibitor plus:
   a. Calcium channel blocker *or*
   b. Alpha-blocker
   c. Central alpha-agonist
   d. Diuretic
5. Diuretic plus:
   a. Any other antihypertensive class
   b. Possible exception: calcium channel blocker (does not usually enhance effects)
6. Beta-blocker plus:
   a. Calcium channel blocker—use caution in the presence of systolic dysfunction or conducting problems, particularly with verapamil or diltiazem.
   b. ACE inhibitor, Ang-II receptor blocker
   c. Diuretic
   d. Alpha-blocker
   e. Do not use with central alpha-agonist because of possible central antagonism and potential for severe withdrawal syndrome
7. Ang-II receptor blocker plus:
   a. Calcium channel blocker
   b. Central alpha-agonist
   c. Alpha-blocker
   d. Diuretic

Combination Antihypertensive Therapy: Selected Drugs: *Summary*

	Calcium Channel Blocker	Alpha-Blocker	Central Alpha-Agonist	Ang-II Blocker/ ACE Inhibitor	Diuretic
Calcium channel blocker		√	√	√	
Alpha-blocker	√		∅	√	√
Central alpha-agonist	√	∅		√	√
Ang II blocker/ ACE inhibitor	√	√	√		√

√, Appropriate combination; ∅, avoid.

Combinations of these *four classes* of antihypertensive drugs in low doses can achieve:

1. Additive or synergistic reduction in blood pressure
2. Reduced adverse effects
3. Improvement of the structural and metabolic components of the hypertension syndrome

Antihypertensive Therapy: Efficacy of Monotherapy

Drug Class	White (%)	African-American (%)	Elderly (%)
Diuretic	50	60	50
Beta-blocker	50	30–40	20–30
Calcium channel blocker	75	75–80	75–80
ACE inhibitor	60	60	60
Alpha-blocker	60	60	60
Central alpha-agonist	60	60	60
Ang-II blocker	60	60	60

Selected Drug Interactions with Antihypertensive Therapy*[116]

Class of Agent	Increase Efficacy	Decrease Efficacy	Effect on Other Drugs
Diuretics	• Diuretics that act at different sites in the nephron (e.g., furosemide + thiazides)	• Resin-binding agents • NSAIDs • Steroids	• Diuretics raise serum lithium levels. • Potassium-sparing agents may exacerbate hyperkalemia due to ACE inhibitors.
Beta-blockers	• Cimetidine (hepatically metabolized beta-blockers) • Quinidine (hepatically metabolized beta-blockers) • Food (hepatically metabolized beta-blockers)	• NSAIDs • Withdrawal of clonidine • Agents that induce rifampin and phenobarbital	• Propranolol hydrochloride induces hepatic enzymes to increase clearance of drugs with similar metabolic pathways. • Beta-blockers may mask and prolong insulin-induced hypoglycemia. • Heart block may occur with nondihydropyridine calcium antagonists. • Sympathomimetics cause unopposed alpha-adrenoceptor-mediated vasoconstriction. • Beta-blockers increase angina-inducing potential of cocaine.
ACE inhibitors	• Chlorpromazine or clozapine	• NSAIDs • Antacids • Food decreases absorption (moexipril)	• ACE inhibitors may raise serum lithium levels. • ACE inhibitors may exacerbate hyperkalemic effect of potassium-sparing diuretics.

Drug class			
Calcium antagonists	• Grapefruit juice (some dihydropyridines) • Cimetidine or ranitidine (hepatically metabolized calcium antagonists)	• Agents that induce hepatic enzymes, including rifampin and phenobarbital	• Cyclosporine levels increase† with diltiazem hydrochloride, verapamil hydrochloride, mibefradil dihydrochloride, or nicardipine hydrochloride (but not felodipine, isradipine, or nifedipine). • Nondihydropyridines increase levels of other drugs metabolized by the same hepatic enzyme system, including digoxin, quinidine, sulfonylureas, and theophylline. • Verapamil hydrochloride may lower serum lithium levels.
Alpha-blockers			• Prazosin may decrease clearance of verapamil hydrochloride.
Central alpha₂-agonists and peripheral neuronal blockers	• Tricyclic antidepressants (and probably phenothiazines) • Monoamine oxidase inhibitors • Sympathomimetics or phenothiazines antagonize guanethidine monosulfate or guanadrel sulfate • Iron salts may reduce methyldopa absorption		• Methyldopa may increase serum lithium levels. • Severity of clonidine hydrochloride withdrawal may be increased by beta-blockers. • Many agents used in anesthesia are potentiated by clonidine hydrochloride.

*Reproduced with permission from Joint National Committee on Prevention, Detection, Evaluation, and Treatment of High Blood Pressure. The Sixth Report of the Joint National Committee on Prevention, Detection, Evaluation, and Treatment of High Blood Pressure. Arch Intern Med. 1997;157:2413–2446.

Maximum Recommended Doses* of Antihypertensive Drugs with Best Treatment Characteristics

	Dose/Day (mg)
Calcium channel blockers	
Amlodipine (Norvasc)	10
Diltiazem (Cardizem SR and CD, Dilacor XR, Tiazac)	480
Felodipine (Plendil)	10
Isradipine (DynaCirc)	10
Nicardipine (Cardene and Cardene SR)	120
Nifedipine (Adalat Oros and CC, Procardia XL)	90
Nisoldipine (Sular)	60
Verapamil (Calan SR, Isoptin SR, Verelan, Covera HS)	480
ACE inhibitors	
Benazepril (Lotensin)	40
Captopril (Capoten)	50
Enalapril (Vasotec)	40
Fosinopril (Monopril)	80
Lisinopril (Prinivil, Zestril)	40
Moexipril (Univasc)	30
Quinapril (Accupril)	80
Ramipril (Altace)	20
Trandolapril (Mavik)	4
Perindopril (Aceon)	16
Central alpha-agonists	
Clonidine (Catapres and Catapres-TTS)	0.3/TTS-3
Guanabenz (Wytensin)	16
Guanfacine (Tenex)	2
Alpha-blockers	
Doxazosin (Cardura)	10
Prazosin (Minipress)	10
Terazosin (Hytrin)	10
Other	
Indapamide (Lozol)	2.5
Angiotensin II blockers	
Losartan (Cozaar)	100
Valsartan (Diovan)	160
Irbesartan (Avapro)	300
Telmisartan (Micardis)	80
Candesartan cilexetil (Atacand)	32
Eprosartan (Teveten)	600

*Approximately 80% to 90% of total antihypertensive effect achieved in most patients.

Diuretics[103–105]

The mechanism of action of diuretics is inhibition of NaCl resorption in the renal tubules. There is an initial reduction in CO secondary to reduction in plasma volume and extracellular fluid volume, but SVR is reduced with long-term therapy (after 4 to 8 weeks).

Diuretics are used as monotherapy to treat mild to moderate hypertension or as an adjunct to other antihypertensives. The best clinical use is in patients with volume-dependent (low-renin) hypertension or normal-renin hypertension and in African-Americans. The major differences among the diuretics are related to duration and site of action as well as potency of diuretic action. The adverse effects are similar, particularly among the thiazide diuretics. *Lower doses* of diuretics (i.e., HCTZ 12.5 to 25 mg/day or its equivalent) are now recommended for treatment of essential hypertension during the initial treatment period; the dose is then adjusted as necessary. The maximum antihypertensive dose should not exceed 50 mg of HCTZ or its equivalent. Approximately 80% of the antihypertensive effect of HCTZ is achieved with a 12.5 mg/day dose; 95% is achieved with a 25 mg/day dose.[105] Therefore, there is a relatively flat dose-response curve for the *antihypertensive efficacy* of thiazide diuretics, whereas the *diuretic effect* may continue up to doses of 100 mg/day of HCTZ.

Indapamide offers many advantages over other diuretics, which may make it the diuretic of choice in treating hypertension.[106,107] Indapamide has a better metabolic profile (lipid neutral, no glucose intolerance, and less effect on potassium and magnesium). It reduces LVH and platelet aggregation. There is no effect on insulin resistance. Indapamide is also effective in the presence of renal insufficiency.

1. *Classification:* Diuretic inhibition of NaCl resorption in renal tubules.
2. *Mechanism:*
   a. Initial reduction in CO secondary to reduction in plasma volume and extracellular fluid volume.
   b. Long-term reduction in SVR.
   c. Direct vasodilator action.

89

3. *Pharmacology:* See individual diuretics listings.
4. *Hemodynamics:*
   a. MAP reduced.
   b. CO slightly reduced (1%–5%).
   c. SVR reduced.
   d. HR increased.
   e. RBF, RPF, and GFR slightly reduced.
   f. Renin, aldosterone, and angiotensin II increased.
   g. Postural hypotension (mild).
5. *Clinical use:*
   a. Monotherapy, initial therapy in mild to moderate hypertension.
   b. Adjunctive with other antihypertensives.
   c. Relatively inexpensive.
   d. Reduces supine and upright BP.
   e. Fairly well tolerated.
   f. No tachyphylaxis.
   g. Best in volume-dependent (low-renin) hypertension, normal-renin hypertension, African-Americans.
6. *Major differences in diuretics:*
   a. Duration and site of action.
   b. Potency of diuretic action (loop diuretics > thiazides).
   c. Efficacy with renal insufficiency (loop > metolazone > indapamide > thiazides).
   d. Efficacy on BP control (thiazides > loop).
   e. Hemodynamic regulatory mechanisms.
   f. Hormonal regulatory mechanisms.
7. *Most common adverse effects:*
   a. Hypokalemia.
   b. Hypomagnesemia.
   c. Hyperuricemia.
   d. Hyperglycemia (less with loop diuretics).
   e. Hyponatremia.
   f. Hypochloremia.
   g. Hyperlipidemia (mostly thiazides) including hypertriglyceridemia, hypercholesterolemia, increased LDL cholesterol, decreased HDL cholesterol.

    h. Azotemia.

    i. Hypercalcemia (usually only thiazide-like diuretics).

    j. Impotence—20%–25% of male patients.

    k. Dermatologic reactions, rash, purpura.

    l. Blood dyscrasias.

    m. Cardiac arrhythmias.

    n. Volume depletion and postural hypotension.

    o. Metabolic alkalosis.

    p. Hyperreninemia.

    q. Hyperaldosteronism (secondary).

    r. Pancreatitis.

    s. Allergic disorders.

    t. Vasculitis.

8. *Contraindications:*

    a. Anuria.

    b. Known allergy (some sulfa-allergic patients).

9. *Dose and tablet strength:*

    a. Start with a low dose (12.5 mg of HCTZ or equivalent) to control BP, and titrate dose up to a maximum of 25 mg/day of HCTZ or equivalent. Higher doses are more effective in volume-dependent, low-renin hypertension; 95% of patients respond to 25mg/day.

    b. For treatment of hypertension, but not for the diuretic effect, there is a *flat dose response* over 25 mg/day of HCTZ or its equivalent.

    c. HCTZ and other thiazides are not effective if the creatinine clearance is less than 35 mL/min.

    d. Indapamide offers many advantages over other diuretics.

Diuretics Highlights*

	Preparation	Mechanism of Action	Pharmacodynamics
Thiazides (benzothiadiazine derivatives)			
Chlorothiazide (Diuril)—Merck	250 mg 500 mg	See HCTZ	Duration: 6–12 hr
Cyclothiazide (Anhydron)—Lilly	2 mg	See HCTZ	Duration: 12 hr
HCTZ (Oretic)—Abbott (Esidrix)—Novartis (Hydro-DIURIL)—Merck	25–50 mg 25–50 mg 25–100 mg	Inhibits resorption of NaCl and thereby increases the quantity of Na^1 traversing the distal tubule and volume of water excreted. Initial antihypertensive effect is due to volume contraction and lower CO. Long-term antihypertensive effect due to lower SVR.	Duration: 6–12 hr

Hemodynamics	Adverse Effects	Contra-indications	Daily Dosage	Drug Interactions
See HCTZ	See HCTZ	See HCTZ	250–500 mg	See HCTZ
See HCTZ	See HCTZ	See HCTZ	1–2 mg on alternate days	See HCTZ
MAP reduced CO slightly reduced initially Plasma volume reduced SVR decreased HR increased NE increased Aldosterone increased PRA increased Angiotensin II increased	Hyponatremia Hypokalemia Hyperuricemia Hypercalcemia Hyperglycemia Hypomagnesemia Hypochloremia Metabolic alkalosis Volume depletion Postural hypotension Hyperlipidemia Increased total cholesterol, triglycerides Decreased HDL Increased LDL	Anuria Hypertensitivity to sulfona-milde derivatives	6.25–50 mg	Cholestyramine: decreased thiazide effect Corticosteroids: increased potassium loss Diazoxide: increased hyperglycemic effect Digitalis glycosides: increased digitalis toxicity (hypokalemia and hypomagnesemia) Indomethacin: decreased antihypertensive and natriuretic effects NSAIDs: decreased diuretic and antihypertensive effects

	Preparation	Mechanism of Action	Pharmacodynamics
Methyclothiazide (Enduron)—Abbott	2.5 mg 5 mg	See HCTZ	Duration: 24 hr Peak: 2 hr
Polythiazide (Renese)—Pfizer	1 mg 2 mg	See HCTZ Increases excretion of Na^+ and H_2O	Duration: 24–48 hr
Chlorthalidone (Hygroton)— Rhône-Poulenc Rorer (Thalitone)—BI	4 mg 25 mg 50 mg 100 mg 25 mg	Site of action is at the cortical diluting segment of the distal tubule	Duration: 24–72 hr Onset: 2 hr
Loop diuretics	Oral: 0.5 mg, 1 mg	Decreases chloride and secondary	Onset: ½ hr
Bumetanide (Bumex)—Roche	IV: 0.25 mg/mL	sodium resorption in ascending limb of the loop of Henle	Peak: 1–1½ hr Half-life: 4–6 hr Metabolism: liver Excretion: renal
Ethacrynic acid (Edecrin)—Merck	25 mg 50 mg IV powder: 50 mg diluted to 100 mL	See Furosemide	Duration: 1–4 hr Onset: 1 hr
Torsemide (Demadex)— Boehringer Mannheim	5 mg 10 mg 20 mg 100 mg IV: 2 mL (20 mg) vial IV: 5 mL (10 mg/mL) vial	See Furosemide	Onset: ½ hr— simultaneous food intake delays absorption Peak: 1 hr Half-life: 3.5 hr Metabolism: liver Excretion: renal Less protein bound

Hemodynamics	Adverse Effects	Contra-indications	Daily Dosage	Drug Interactions
See HCTZ	See HCTZ	Renal decompensation Hypersensitivity	2.5–5 mg	See HCTZ
See HCTZ	See HCTZ	See HCTZ	1–4 mg	See HCTZ
See Thiazides	Hypomagnesemia Increases cholesterol, triglycerides, and LDL Decreases HDL	See HCTZ	12.5–50 mg	See Thiazides
GFR, RPF, RBF preserved Reduction in free water clearance	Hypokalemia Hypochloremic alkalosis Hyperuricemia Ototoxicity Muscle pain and tenderness Dizziness Hypotension Weakness	See HCTZ	Average dose: 1–2 mg Range: 0.5–10 mg Maximum: 10 mg	Probenecid: reduces bumetanide effectiveness Indomethacin: blunts sodium excretion associated with bumetanide Lithium: reduces renal clearance of bumetanide, high risk of lithium toxicity
See Furosemide	Gastrointestinal symptoms common with larger doses Hyperuricemia	Anuria	50–100 mg Should not exceed 400 mg	Oral anticoagulants: increased anticoagulant effect Aminoglycoside antibiotics, digitalis: see Furosemide
GFR, RPF, RBF acid base balance preserved Increased urinary excretion of sodium chloride + H_2O	Dizziness Headache Nausea Weakness Vomiting Hyperglycemia Excessive urination Hyperuricemia Hypokalemia Excessive thirst	Anuria Hypersensitivity	Intial: 5 mg qd Range: 5–10 mg qd Maximum: 10 mg qd	Salicylates: salicylate toxicity NSAIDs: possible renal dysfunction Indomethacin: blunts sodium excretion associated with torsemide Probenecid: reduces torsemide effectiveness Lithium: reduces renal clearance of torsemide, high risk of torsemide toxicity

	Preparation	Mechanism of Action	Pharmacodynamics
Furosemide	20 mg	Primarily inhibits	Duration: 1–4 hr
(Lasix)—	40 mg	the resorption	Onset: 1 hr
Hoechst Marion Roussel	80 mg	of Cl^-, Na^+,	Peak: 1–2 hr
		and H_2O in the	Metabolism: liver
		ascending loop	Excretion: renal
		of Henle and	
		exerts a weak	
		diuretic effect	
		in the proximal	
		and distal tubules	
Diuretic of the	5 mg	Acts within the	Duration:
pyridine-sulfonyurea	10 mg	lumen of the	oral 6–8 hr
class (Demadex)—	20 mg	thick ascending	IV 6–8 hr
Boehringer Mannheim	100 mg	portion of the	Onset: oral 1 hr
		loop of Henle	IV 10 min
		where it inhibits	Peak: oral 1–2 hr
		the $Na^+/K^+/Cl^-$	IV 1 hr
		carrier system	Excretions:
			hepatic 80%
			renal 20%
			Bioavailability: 80%

Hemodynamics	Adverse Effects	Contra-indications	Daily Dosage	Drug Interactions
Decreased pulmonary wedge pressure (PWP) Decreases CO Decreases SVR	Fluid and electrolyte imbalance Hypomagnesemia Hypokalemia Mild diarrhea Nerve deafness Decreases HDL	Anuria Azotemia	20–150 mg	Digitalis glycosides: increased digitalis toxicity (hypokalemia and hypomagnesemia) Indomethacin: decreased antihypertensive and natriuretic effect Probenecid: decreased diuretic effect NSAIDs: decreased diuretic and antihypertensive effects Aminoglycoside antibiotics: increased ototoxicity and nephrotoxicity
GFR, RPF preserved CO decreased SVR decreased	Fluid and electrolyte imbalance Dizziness Headache Excessive urination Rhinitis Nausea	Known sensitivity to Demadex or to sulfonylurea Use with caution: Hepatic disease with cirrhosis and ascites Ototoxicity Volume and electrolyte depletion	Hypertension: Initial dose 5 mg qd Increase to 10 mg qd if inadequate BP response after 4–6 weeks Maximum recommended: 10 mg qd	Indomethacin: natriuretic effects partially inhibited Lithium: may decrease renal clearance Salicylates: salicylate toxicity Cholestyramine: decreases the absorption of oral Demadex

	Preparation	Mechanism of Action	Pharmacodynamics
Potassium-sparing diuretics			
Amiloride (Midamor)—Merck	5 mg	Inhibits K^+/Na^+ exchange in the distal tubule—a weak diuretic antihypertensive	Duration: 24 hr Onset: 2 hr Peak: 6–10 hr Excretion: kidney
Spironolactone (Aldactone)—Searle	25 mg 50 mg 100 mg	Antagonist of aldosterone through competitive binding of receptors at the aldosterone-dependent Na^+/K^+ exchange site in the distal convoluted renal tubule; causes an increase in Na^+ and water excreted	Duration: 12–48 hr
Triamterene (Dyrenium)—SmithKline Beecham	50 mg 100 mg	Not a diuretic but has a diuretic effect on the distal renal tubules, inhibiting the resorption of Na^+ in exchange for K^+	Duration: 7–9 hr Onset: 2–4 hr

Hemodynamics	Adverse Effects	Contra-indications	Daily Dosage	Drug Interactions
See Thiazides	See Triamterene	Hyperkalemia Should not be used with other potassium-conserving drugs in patients with impaired renal function	5–10 mg Should not exceed 20 mg	NSAIDs: renal failure, hyperkalemia ACE inhibitors: hyperkalemia
See Thiazides	Gynecomastia Menstrual irregularity or amenorrhea Postmenopausal bleeding Hyperkalemia Hyponatremia Gastrointestinal symptoms Impotence Fever Rash	Anuria Acute renal insufficiency Significant impairment of renal function Hyperkalemia	100–400 mg to treat hyper-aldosteronism 50–100 mg to treat essential hypertension	Salicylates: decreased diuretic effect Anticoagulations decreased anticoagulant effect Captopril: hyperkalemia Ether, nitrous oxide: hypotension
See Thiazides	Blood dyscrasias Photosensitivity Skin rash Hyperkalemia Hyperglycemia Metabolic acidosis	Anuria Renal insufficiency Severe hepatic disease	100 mg bid after meals Should not exceed 300 mg	Indomethacin and NSAIDs: renal failure Captopril and ACE inhibitors: hyperkalemia (additive) Ether, nitrous oxide: hypotension (additive)

	Preparation	Mechanism of Action	Pharmacodynamics
Combination diuretics			
HCTZ 50 mg + amiloride 5 mg (Moduretic) — Merck	Combination tablet only	Amiloride is a K^+-conserving diuretic with weak, natriuretic antihypertensive activity. HCTZ blocks the resorption of Na^+ and K^+, thereby increasing the quantity of Na^+ traversing the distal tubule and the volume of water excreted	Duration: 24 hr Onset: 1–2 hr
HCTZ 25 mg + spironolactone 25 mg (Aldactazide) — Searle	Combination tablet only	Combination of diuretic agents with different but complementary mechanisms and sites of action, providing additive diuretic and anti-hypertensive effects and preserving K^+	Duration: 24 hr Onset: 1–2 hr
HCTZ 25 mg + Triamterene 50 mg (Dyazide) — SmithKline Beecham	Combination capsule only	HCTZ blocks resorption of Na^+ and Cl^- and thereby increases the quantity of Na^+ traversing the distal tubule and volume of water excreted. Triamterene has a weak diuretic effect on the distal renal tubules, inhibiting the resorption of Na^+ in exchange for K^+	Duration: 7–9 hr

Hemodynamics	Adverse Effects	Contra-indications	Daily Dosage	Drug Interactions
See Thiazides	Electrolye imbalance Elevates BUN Hyperkalemia Mild skin rash	Renal impairment Patients receiving K⁺-conserving agents Hyperkalemia	1–2 tablets	See HCTZ and Amiloride
See Thiazides	Gynecomastia Gastrointestinal symptoms Hyperkalemia Rash	Anuria Acute renal insufficiency Acute, severe hepatic failure Hyperkalemia	Optimal dosage established by individual titration of the components	See HCTZ and Spironolactone
Reduces SVR Mild reduction in CO Mild reduction in plasma volume (See Thiazides)	Electrolye imbalance Muscle cramps Rash Weakness Photosensitivity Gastrointestinal disturbances	Renal dysfunction Azotemia Hyperkalemia Anuria	1–2 capsules Not to exceed 4 capsules†	See HCTZ and Triamterene

	Preparation	Mechanism of Action	Pharmacodynamics

HCTZ
  50 mg
  +
Triamterene
  75 mg (Maxzide)—
  Lederle
	Tablet (scored)	HCTZ blocks NaCl
		  resorption and
		  later reduces SVR.
		  Triamterene has
		  a weak diuretic
		  effect on distal
		  renal rubule,
		  preserves K$^+$
			Duration: 6–12 hr
			Onset: 2 hr
			Peak: 4 hr
			Excretion: kidney
			Improved bioavailabili
			  over Dyazide

Quinazoline
  diuretic
  derivative
  Metolazone
  (Zaroxolyn)—Fisons
  (Diulo)—Searle
	
	2.5 mg
	5 mg
	10 mg
		Acts primarily to
		  inhibit Na$^+$
		  resorption at the
		  cortical diluting
		  site and in the
		  proximal convo-
		  luted tubule
			Duration: 12–24 hr
			Onset: 1 hr
			Peak: 24 hr
			Excretion: renal

Indoline
  diuretic
  derivative
  Indapamide
  (Lozol)—Rhône-Poulenc
    Rorer
	2.5 mg
	5 mg
		Similar to thiazides—
		  acts on the cortical
		  diluting segment;
		  may be effective
		  in mild renal
		  insufficiency
			Duration: 24 hr
			Onset: 1 hr
			Peak: 2 hr
			Metabolism: liver
			Excretion:
			  renal 70%
			  bile 23%

*Consult the *Physicians' Desk Reference* for full prescribing information.
†Bioequivalence is low, with only 30% absorption.
‡Bioequivalence is improved compared with Dyazide; 60% absorption.

Hemodynamics	Adverse Effects	Contra-indications	Daily Dosage	Drug Interactions
Reduces SVR Mild reduction in CO Mild reduction in plasma volume (See Thiazides)	Electrolyte imbalance Muscle cramps Rash Weakness Photosentivity Gastrointestinal disturbances	Renal dysfunction Azotemia Hyperkalemia Anuria	½ to 1 tablet‡	See HCTZ and Triamterene
See Thiazides	Azotemia Hyperglycemia Hyperuricemia Hypercalcemia Hyponatremia Hypokalemia Hypomagnesemia	Renal insufficiency	2.5–5 mg Higher doses may be indicated with other disorders	See Thiazides
MAP reduced CO reduced SVR reduced Minimal change in RBF, RPF, GFR	Hypokalemia Hypomagnesemia Hyperuricemia Hyponatremia Hypochloremia	See Thiazides	Average: 2.5–5 mg Maximum: 5 mg	See Thiazides

Central Alpha-Agonists[103,104]

The central alpha-agonists all stimulate the central postsynaptic alpha$_2$ receptor in the brain stem, which reduces sympathetic nervous system activity to the periphery. This results in a reduction in SVR, plasma and urine NE levels, and PRA. CO, RBF, and GFR are preserved at rest and with exercise.

Common side effects are sedation and dry mouth, which are minimal with low-dose long-term therapy. Concern about withdrawal syndrome has been overemphasized with all these drugs, particularly clonidine. When low doses are used, the frequency of withdrawal syndrome is minimal and probably less than that with beta-blockers.

Antihypertensive efficacy is excellent and similar with all of the central alpha-agonists. Selection of therapy depends more on some of the unique side effects, duration of action, and cost.

Clonidine, guanabenz, and guanfacine all have a neutral or favorable effect on serum lipids and glucose compared with methyldopa, which has an unfavorable effect. Methyldopa reduces HDL cholesterol and increases triglycerides. There is little reason to use methyldopa now because as the side effects are greater than and efficacy is inferior to those of the other central alpha-agonists.[108–110]

1. Clonidine (Catapres): oral and transdermal patch
2. Guanabenz (Wytensin)
3. Guanfacine (Tenex)
4. Methyldopa (Aldomet)

Alpha Receptors

Alpha receptors are primarily of two types:

1. *Presynaptic (prejunctional):* located at the membranes of the neurons that contain the neurotransmitter NE. Stimulation inhibits the release of NE from the postganglionic sympathetic nerve ending. NE in the synaptic cleft inhibits its own release.
2. *Postsynaptic:* located on the target organ. Activation results in an agonist effect (vasoconstriction in the periphery) but reduced sympathetic activity centrally.

Central Alpha-Agonists: Similarities

1. Stimulation of central postsynaptic alpha$_2$ receptors in the nucleus tractus solitarii of the medulla oblongata results in:
   a. Reduced sympathetic nervous system activity.
   b. Reduced NE levels in serum and urine.
   c. Reduced PRA owing to reduced NE levels.
   d. Increased vagal stimulation (bradycardia):
      (1) Clonidine: direct.
      (2) Guanabenz: direct.
      (3) Guanfacine: direct.
      (4) Methyldopa: indirect (alpha-methylnorepinephrine).
2. Peripheral alpha agonist pressor response is overwhelmed by central alpha-agonist effect except rarely with:
   a. Intravenous doses (transient pressor effects).
   b. High oral doses.
3. Peripheral sympathetic reflexes remain intact, so fewer problems occur with:
   a. Postural hypotension: methyldopa effect greater than that of clonidine, guanabenz, guanfacine.
   b. Exercise: preserved with all four drugs.
   c. Sexual dysfunction: methyldopa effect greater than that of clonidine, guanabenz, or guanfacine.
4. Lowering of BP is not associated with reduction of systemic or regional blood flow.
5. Minimal to no sodium or water retention or weight gain occurs except with methyldopa. Natriuresis occurs in some patients with clonidine, guanabenz, and guanfacine.
6. Hemodynamic effects are similar.
7. Drugs are effective as monotherapy.
8. Adjunctive therapy with other antihypertensive drugs allows for additive or synergistic effects at lower doses of each drug. The recommended average maximum is:
   a. Clonidine: 0.4 mg (oral); TTS—0.3 mg/day.
   b. Guanabenz: 16 to 24 mg/day.
   c. Guanfacine: 2 mg/day.
   d. Methyldopa: 2000 mg/day.
9. Dose equivalency: Clonidine 0.1 mg = guanabenz 4 mg = guanfacine 0.25 mg = methyldopa 250 to 500 mg.

Central Alpha-Agonists Highlights*

	Preparation	Mechanism of Action	Pharmacodynamics
Clonidine (Catapres)— Boehringer Ingelheim	0.1 mg (oral) 0.2 mg (oral) 0.3 mg (oral) TTS 1–3	Selective stimulation of postsynaptic alpha$_2$ adrenergic receptors in depressor site of vasomotor center of medulla, nucleus tractus solitarii, and hypothalamus. Reduces efferent sympathetic tone and increases vagal tone to heart, peripheral vasculature, and kidney. Reduces SVR, causing vasodilation and lowering blood pressure. Spares peripheral reflexes. Reduces PRA	Onset: ½–1 hr Peak: 3–5 hr Plasma half-life: 12–16 hr Metabolism: liver (minimal) Excretion: renal TTS—duration of antihypertensive effect: 1 week

Hemodynamics	Adverse Effects	Contra-indications	Daily Dosage	Drug Interactions
MAP reduced	Sedation and drowsiness	Sick sinus syndrome	Initial: 0.1 mg hs and increase by 0.1 mg q 3–4 days, giving larger bid doses at bedtime. Some qd, usually bid	Tricyclic anti-depressants and beta-adrenergic blockers: loss of antihypertensive effect in some patients
CO unchanged	Dry mouth	Second-or third-degree AV block		
HR reduced (10%)	Dizziness			
SVR reduced	Withdrawal syndrome and rebound hypertension (uncommon with doses <1.2 mg qd)			
RBF, RPF, GFR: no change or increase				
RVR reduced				
Plasma and urinary NE and EPI reduced				
Angiotensin II reduced	Weakness		Average: 0.4–0.6 mg	
PRA reduced	Headache		Maximum: 1.2 mg	
Aldosterone reduced	Bradycardia		Range: 0.2–1.2 mg	
Exercise response preserved	Constipation		TTS: once per week	
PWP reduced	Impotence (uncommon—4%)		TTS—1, 2, or 3	
Fluid retention: minimal to none				
Diuresis in some patients				

	Preparation	Mechanism of Action	Pharmacodynamics
Guanabenz (Wytensin) — Wyeth-Ayerst	4 mg 8 mg	Stimulation of post-synaptic alpha$_2$ receptors in medulla reduces sympathetic activity and reduces SVR and PRA	Onset: 1 hr Peak: 4 hr Plasma and half-life: 6 hr Metabolism: 75% (site undetermined) Excretion: renal: 80%
Guanfacine (Tenex) — A.H. Robins	1 mg 2 mg	Reduces sympathetic tone, SVR, and HR	Onset: 1 hr Peak: 4 hr Plasma half-life: 12 hr Excretion: renal

Hemodynamics	Adverse Effects	Contra-indications	Daily Dosage	Drug Interactions
MAP reduced	Dry mouth	Pregnancy	Average dose: 16 mg	Potentiates central nervous system depressant drugs
CO unchanged	Sedation and drowsiness		Range: 8–48 mg	
HR reduced (minimal)	Fatigue		Maximum: 48 mg	
SVR reduced	Impotence			
RBF, RPF, GFR: no change	Withdrawal syndrome			
RVR reduced	Rebound and overshoot hypertension			
Plasma and urinary NE and EPI reduced	Dizziness			
Aldosterone reduced	Weakness			
PRA reduced	Headache			
Angiotensin II reduced	Constipation			
Exercise response preserved				
Plasma volume: unchanged				
Diuresis in some patients				
MAP reduced	See Clonidine	Allergy to guanfacine	1 mg hs	See Clonidine
CO unchanged			Maximum: 3 mg hs	
HR reduced (10%)				
SVR reduced				
RBF, RPF, GFR: no change or increase				
RVR reduced				
Plasma and urinary NE and EPI reduced				
Angiotensin II reduced				
PRA reduced				
Aldosterone reduced				
Exercise response preserved				
PWP reduced				
Fluid retention: minimal to none				
Diuresis in some patients				

	Preparation	Mechanism of Action	Pharmacodynamics
Methyldopa (Aldomet)— Merck	125 mg 250 mg 500 mg Also available in elixir, 250 mg/mL	Alpha-methylnorepi-nephrine stimulates a postsynaptic alpha$_2$ adrenergic receptor in the medulla and decreases sympathetic outflow, which reduces SVR and PRA. Also has some peripheral action	Onset: 2–3 hr Peak: 5 hr Plasma half-life: 12 hr Metabolism: hepatic Excretion: renal

*Consult the *Physicians' Desk Reference* for full prescribing information.
†Variable oral absorption, 50%–80%.

Hemodynamics	Adverse Effects	Contra-indications	Daily Dosage	Drug Interactions
MAP reduced	Lassitude	Active hepatic disease	Average: 250–3000 mg bid schedule	Beta-adrenergic blockers: loss of antihypertensive action in some patients
CO unchanged or some decrease	Drowsiness and sedation		Maximum: 3000 mg†	
HR slightly decreased	Dry mouth			
SVR decreased	Mild orthostasis			Oral contraceptives: decreased antihypertensive effect
RBF, RPR, GRF: no change	Positive Coombs' test and anemia			
RVR reduced	Positive rheumatoid factor and lupus erythematosus preparation			
Angiotensin II reduced				
PRA reduced	Impotence			
Aldosterone reduced	Hepatitis			
Exercise response preserved	Withdrawal syndrome			
Plasma volume increased	Rebound and overshoot hypertension			
	Altered mental acuity			
	Depression			

Comparison of Commonly Used Oral Central Alpha-Agonists

Drug	Initial Dose (mg)	Range of Usual Total Daily Dose (mg)	Orthostasis	Effect on RBF and GFR	Fluid Retention	CO	HR	Effect on Plasma Renin	Insufficiency States Needing Dose Change	Available Tablet/Capsule Sizes (mg)
Clonidine	0.1 bid	0.2–1.2	Rare	→/↑	Minimal or none	↑	↓	→	Renal insufficiency	0.1, 0.2, 0.3, and TTS 1, 2, 3
Guanabenz	4 bid	8–48	Rare	↑	Minimal or none	↑	→/↓	→	Renal insufficiency	4, 8
Guanfacine	1 hs	1–3	Rare	→/↑	Minimal or none	↑	→/↓	→	Renal insufficiency	1, 2
Methyldopa	250 bid	250–3000	Yes (mild)	↑	Yes	→/↓	→/↓	→	Renal and hepatic insufficiency	125, 250, 500

↑ Increased; ↓ decreased; → no change.

Postganglionic Neuron Inhibitors[103,104]

The postganglionic neuron inhibitors act by depleting catecholamine stores or inhibiting the release of catecholamines in peripheral sympathetic nerve endings. The onset of action is slow except for guanadrel, and the drugs have a long half-life. This class of antihypertensive drugs is best *avoided* unless it is necessary to treat severe refractory hypertension unresponsive to all other medications. The adverse effects are similar, and they are poorly tolerated by most patients.

Postganglionic Neuron Inhibitors Highlights*

	Preparation (mg)	Mechanism of Action	Pharmaco-dynamics	Hemo-dynamics
Guanadrel (Hylorel)— Fisons	10 25	Decreases adrenergic neuronal activity by inhibiting NE release and depleting NE stores in the peripheral nerve endings. Does not cross into central nervous system	Duration: 10–14 hr Peak: 4–6 hr Excretion: renal Metabolism: hepatic Onset: 2 hr	CO reduced Venous capacitance increased SVR reduced Marked Na+ and H_2O retention
Guanethidine (Ismelin)— Novartis	10 25	Interferes with release of NE from sympathetic nerve terminals	Onset: 5–7 days Half-life: 7–14 days Excretion: renal	CO reduced Venous capacitance increased SVR reduced GFR, RBF, RPF reduced Severe NA+ and H_2O retention

Adverse Effects	Contraindications	Daily Dosage (mg)	Drug Interactions
Faintness Orthostatic hypotension Diarrhea Severe volume retention	Avoid use in CHF, angina, cerebro-vascular disease	5–50 mg in divided doses	Tricyclic antidepressants: decreased antihy-pertensive effect Sympathomimetic amines: de-creased antihy-pertensive effect Antihistamines: hypertensive response
False-negative urine vanillylmandelic acid (VMA) and catecholamines Orthostatic and postexertional hypotension Severe Na+ and H₂O retention Impotence Retrograde ejacu-lation Bradycardia CHF Exacerbates angina Diarrhea	Pheochromocytoma Simultaneous use of EPI	10–25 Maximum: 100	Tricyclic anti-depressants: decreased antihy-pertensive effect Oral contraceptives: decreased guanethidine effect Minoxidil: severe orthostatic hypotension Phenothiazines: decreased antihy-pertensive effect Sympathomimetic amines: decreased anti-hypertensive effect Hypoglycemia drugs: enhanced hypoglycemic effect

	Preparation (mg)	Mechanism of Action	Pharmaco-dynamics	Hemo-dynamics
Reserpine	0.1 0.25 1	Depletes catechola-mine stores in both peripheral sympathetic ner-vous system and central nervous system	Onset: 4–6 weeks Half-life: 7 days or more	Bradycardia CO reduced SVR reduced

*Consult the *Physicians' Desk Reference* for full prescribing information.

Adverse Effects	Contraindications	Daily Dosage (mg)	Drug Interactions
False-negative VMA and urine catecholamines	History of or current depression	0.1–0.25 Maximum: 0.25	May prolong or inhibit effects of sympathomimetic amines
Bradycardia	Active peptic ulcer		
Premature ventricular contractions	Hypotension		
Nasal congestion			
Depression			
Na+ and H$_2$O retention			
Postural hypotension			
Weight gain			
Nightmares			
Extrapyramidal reactions			
Lowers HDL cholesterol			

Beta-Blockers—General[103,104]

1. Proposed mechanisms of action in hypertension:
   a. Slowing of heart rate with reduction of CO.
   b. Reduction of cardiac contractility and CO.
   c. Block of renal renin release.
   d. Sympathetic outflow reduced because of central beta effect.
   e. Blockade of postsynaptic peripheral beta receptors.
   f. Competitive antagonism of catecholamines at receptor site.
   g. Increased prostaglandin levels in vascular tissue (indomethacin blocks).
   h. Increased baroreflex sensitivity.
2. At equipotent doses, there is little or no difference in *antihypertensive* effect among the various beta-blockers, and side effects are similar.
3. Antihypertensive efficacy depends on patient profile:
   a. Age: not as effective in the elderly (reduced beta receptors).
   b. Race: not as effective in African-Americans (low renin, volume dependent).
   c. Renin status: best in high-renin and normal-renin patients; not as effective in low-renin patients.
   d. Duration of hypertension:
      (1) Recent onset, younger patient—hyperdynamic with relatively increased CO and relatively increased SVR: possibly effective.
      (2) Established—hypodynamic with reduced CO and elevated SVR: less effective.
4. Antihypertensive effect correlates poorly with plasma levels.
5. All beta-blockers without ISA increase SVR and decrease CO, which is the *opposite* hemodynamic effect desired to reduce BP.

118

Beta-Blockers and Beta Receptors

Beta₁ stimulation:
1. Cardiac stimulation: increased myocardial contractility, stroke volume, and CO; tachycardia; increased AV conduction and automaticity
2. Renin release from kidneys
3. Lipolysis of free fatty acids

Beta₂ stimulation:
1. Bronchodilation
2. Vasodilation
3. Glycogenolysis (liver, skeletal muscle) and lactate production
4. Pancreatic insulin release
5. Smooth muscle relaxation (uterus)
6. Skeletal muscle stimulation: tremor

Beta₁ blockade:
1. Reduction in myocardial contractility and CO
2. Bradycardia and heart block, depressed automaticity
3. Decreased renin release
4. Reduced release of free fatty acids

Beta₂ blockade:
1. Bronchoconstriction
2. Vasoconstriction
3. Abnormal glucose metabolism (liver, skeletal muscle glycogenolysis reduced)
4. Hyperglycemia (inhibited pancreatic insulin release)
5. Smooth muscle contraction (uterus)
6. Skeletal muscle: reduced tremor

Beta-blockers differ mainly in seven properties:
1. Cardioselectivity
2. ISA
3. Membrane-stabilizing activity (MSA)
4. Lipid solubility versus water solubility
5. Pharmacokinetics

6. Potency
7. Platelet aggregation effect

Beta-Blockers: Selectivity

1. *Nonselective:* blockade of both $beta_1$ and $beta_2$ receptors.
   Nadolol
   Penbutolol
   Pindolol
   Propranolol
   Timolol
2. *Cardioselective:* blockade of $beta_1$ receptor with *relative* sparing of blockade of $beta_2$ receptor (susceptible to stimulation by EPI). Cardioselectivity *diminishes* with *increasing doses.*
   Acebutolol
   Atenolol
   Metoprolol
   Betaxolol
   Bisoprolol
3. *ISA:*
   Acebutolol
   Pindolol
   Penbutolol
   Carteolol
4. *Alpha and beta blockade:*
   Labetalol
   Carvedilol

Side Effects and Contraindications of Beta-Blockers[103,104]

Contraindications

1. Sinus bradycardia.
2. Heart block greater than first degree.
3. Cardiogenic shock.
4. Overt cardiac failure.
5. Bronchial asthma/chronic obstructive pulmonary disease.
6. Known hypertensitivity to product.

Side Effects

1. Myocardial depression: CHF, reduced CO (less with drugs with ISA), dyspnea.
2. Bradycardia and heart block (electrical depression) (less with drugs with ISA).
3. Central nervous system (due to penetration of blood-brain barrier): fatigue, lethargy, poor memory, weakness, drowsiness, emotional lability, mental depression, paresthesias, disorientation, hallucinations, psychosis, delirium, catatonia, insomnia, nightmares, dreams, headache, dizziness, vertigo.
4. Gastrointestinal: nausea, diarrhea, constipation, pain, flatulence, ischemic colitis.
5. Respiratory: bronchospasm, wheezing, exacerbation of asthma and chronic obstructive pulmonary disease.
6. Perpheral vascular constriction: Raynaud's phenomenon, claudication, cold extremities (less with pindolol and acebutolol).
7. Inhibition of glycogenolysis.
8. Withdrawal syndrome: severe hypertension, unstable angina, arrhythmias, MI, death.
9. Drug interactions: indomethacin blocks antihypertensive action.

10. Hyperglycemia: exacerbated diabetes mellitus, inhibited insulin release.
11. Hypertriglyceridemia: HDL cholesterol decreased, LDL cholesterol increased, HDL/LDL ratio decreased (except for drugs with ISA).
12. Hypertriglyceridemia: additive with thiazides.
13. Muscle fatigue and exercise-induced fatigue.
14. Impotence and decreased libido.
15. Postural hypotension.
16. Hyperuricemia: additive with thiazides.
17. Hyperkalemia (blocks intracellular transport of K^+).
18. Hyperthyroidism symptoms after sudden withdrawal.
19. Hypoglycemia in:
    a. Diabetes mellitus: masked and prolonged symptoms.
    b. Postanesthesia.
    c. Dialysis.
    d. Fasting (children).
    e. Prolonged exercise.
20. Severe hypertensive response in hypoglycemic patients on beta blockade.
21. Crosses placenta (fetal bradycardia, hypotension, and hypoglycemia).
22. Precipitates labor by increasing uterine contractions in eclampsia.
23. Paradoxic hypertension in presence of catecholamine excess owing to EPI, pheochromocytoma, hypoglycemia, withdrawal of central alpha-agonist during combined therapy, or volume-dependent hypertension.
24. Reduction in GFR, RBF, RPF, which may persist for 6 months to 1 year or longer after discontinuing therapy.
25. Reduced birth weight (atenolol)

Drug Interactions with Beta-Blockers

Interacting Drugs	Adverse Effect
Alcohol	Signs of delirium tremens may be blocked
Barbiturates	Decreased beta-blocker effect
Chlorpromazine	Increased effects of both drugs
Cimetidine	Increased beta-blocker effect
Clonidine	Paradoxic hypertension
Contraceptives, oral	Increased metoprolol and possibly propranolol effect
Diazoxide	Hypotension (additive)
Diltiazem	Cardiac failure
	AV conduction disturbances and sinus bradycardia
Disopyramide	Cardiac failure
Hydralazine	Increased propranolol and metoprolol effects
Hypoglycemics, sulfonylurea	Decreased effect of hypoglycemic agent
	After overdose, prolonged hypoglycemia and decreased glycogenolysis (blocked beta effects of EPI); beta receptor blockade masks tachycardia and tremor during hypoglycemia
Indomethacin	Decreased antihypertensive effect
Insulin	With overdose, prolonged hypoglycemia and decreased glycogenolysis (blocked beta effects of EPI); beta receptor blockade masks tachycardia and tremor during hypoglycemia
Lidocaine	Increased lidocaine toxicity with propranolol
Methyldopa	Hypertensive episode
Nicotine	Decreased propranolol effects; vasoconstriction and hypertension
Nifedipine	Cardiac failure—rare
Prazosin	Increased hypotensive effect of first dose of prazosin
Rifampin	Decreased beta-blocker effects
Sympathomimetic amines	Decreased antihypertensive effect; hypertensive reactions
Sympathomimetic bronchodilators	Decreased bronchodilator effects
Theophyllines	Increased theophylline toxicity; reported only with propranolol
Verapamil	Cardiac failure; AV conduction disturbances and sinus bradycardia

Beta-Blockers Highlights*

	Preparation (mg)	Mechanism of Action	Pharmaco-dynamics	Hemo-dynamics
Acebutolol (Sectral)— Wyeth-Ayerst	200 400	Cardioselective beta-adrenergic receptor block with weak ISA and MSA	Onset: ½–1 hr Peak: 2½ hr Half-life: 3–4 hr ISA: 1+ MSA: 1+ Lipid solubility: low (1+) Metabolism: hepatic Excretion: renal	HR, CO, PRA, RPF, RBF, GFR, aldosterone reduced SVR and RVR unchanged MAP reduced Plasma volume increased or no change
Atenolol (Tenormin)— Zeneca	50 100	Beta₁ selective blocking agent without MSA or ISA. Preferential effect not absolute. Higher doses inhibit beta adrenoreceptors located in the bronchial and vascular musculature	Onset: 1 hr Peak: 2–4 hr Half-life: 6–9 hr ISA: none MSA: none Lipid solubility: low (1+), more water soluble Metabolism: minimal, hepatic (10%) Excretion: renal, unchanged	HR, CO, PRA, GFR, RBF, RPF, aldosterone reduced SVR and RVR increased MAP reduced Plasma volume increased

Adverse Effects	Contraindications	Daily Dosage (mg)	Drug Interactions

See separate list of side effects	See separate list of contraindications	Initial: 400
		Average: 600
		Range:
		    200–1200
		Maximum:
		    1200
			See separate list of drug interactions

See separate list of side effects	See separate list of contraindications	Initial: 25–50 Average: 50 Maximum: 100	See separate list of drug interactions

	Preparation (mg)	Mechanism of Action	Pharmaco-dynamics	Hemo-dynamics
Betaxolol (Kerlone)— Searle	10 20	Cardioselective	Onset: 1 hr Peak: 3 hr Half-life: 14–22 hr ISA: none MSA: 1+ Lipid solubility: none Metabolism: hepatic Excretion: renal	HR, CO, PRA, GFR, RBF, RPF, aldo-sterone reduced SVR and RVR increased MAP reduced Plasma volume increased or no change
Metoprolol (Lopressor)— Novartis (Toprol XL)— Astra	50 100	Selective beta-adrenergic blocking agent with relative selectivity for beta adrenore-ceptors located primarily in cardiac muscle. Specificity is lost with large doses	Onset: 1 hr Peak: 1½–2 hr Half-life: 3–4 hr ISA: none MSA: minimal (1+) to none Lipid solubility: moderate (3+) Metabolism: hepatic Excretion: hepatic to renal	HR, CO, PRA, RPF, RBF, GFR, and aldo-sterone reduced SVR and RVR increased MAP reduced Plasma volume increased
Nadolol (Corgard)— Bristol-Myers Squibb	20 40 80 120 160	Nonselective beta-adrenergic re-ceptor antagonist	Onset: 1–2 hr Peak: 3–4 hr Half-life: 20–24 hr ISA: none MSA: none Lipid solubility: low (1+), more water soluble Metabolism: minimal, hepatic (27%) Excretion: renal, unchanged (73%)	HR, CO, PRA, aldosterone reduced May not alter RPF and GFR RVR unchanged SVR increased MAP reduced Plasma volume increased

Adverse Effects	Contraindications	Daily Dosage (mg)	Drug Interactions
See separate list of side effects	See separate list of contraindications	Initial: 10 Average dose: 10 Maximum dose: 20	See separate list of drug interactions
See separate list of side effects	See separate list of contraindications	Initial: 50 (qd or bid) Average: 200 (lose beta selectivity at 150) Range: 50–450 Maximum: 450	See separate list of drug interactions
		Initial: 50–100 qd Maximum: 400	
See separate list of side effects	See separate list of contraindications	Initial: 40 Average: 160 Range: 40–340 Maximum: 340	See separate list of drug interactions

	Preparation (mg)	Mechanism of Action	Pharmaco-dynamics	Hemo-dynamics
Carteolol (Cartrol)-Abbott Laboratories	2.5 5	Nonselective beta-adrenergic receptor antagonist with ISA	Onset: ½–1 hr Peak: 1–3 hr Half-life: 6 hr ISA: yes MSA: none Lipid solubility: low Metabolism: 30–50% hepatic Excretion: renal, unchanged (50–70%)	HR reduced < with other beta blockers (2–5 beats/min) CO reduced < with other beta blockers or not at all MAP reduced Plasma volume increased SVR unchanged or reduced GFR, RBF, RPF preserved or slightly reduce
Penbutolol (Levatol)—Schwartz Pharma	20	Nonselective beta-adrenergic antagonist with mild ISA, mild partial agonist activity	Onset: ½–1 hr Peak: 1½–3 hr Half-life: 5 hr ISA: 0–1 + MSA: none Lipid solubility: low (1+) Metabolism: hepatic Excretion: renal	HR, CO, PRA, aldosterone reduced GFR, RBF, RPF unchange MAP reduced Plasma volume unchanged or increased
Pindolol (Visken)—Novartis	5 10	Nonselective beta-adrenergic antagonist with ISA	Onset: ½–1 hr Peak: 1–2 hr Half-life: 3–4 hr ISA: yes (3+) MSA: minimal (1+) to none Lipid solubility: moderate (3+) Metabolism: hepatic (60%) Excretion: renal (40%)	HR reduced less than with othe beta-blockers (4–8 beats/min) CO reduced less than with othe beta-blockers or not at all SVR unchanged or reduced MAP reduced GFR, RBF, RPF preserved or slightly reduce RVR unchanged or reduced Plasma volume increased

Adverse Effects	Contraindications	Daily Dosage (mg)	Drug Interactions
See separate list of side effects	See separate list of contraindications	Initial: 2.5 Range: 5–10 Maximum: 10	See separate list of drug interactions
See separate list of side effects	See separate list of contraindications	Initial: 10 Average: 20–40 Maximum: 50	See separate list of drug interactions
Neutral effects on lipids See separate list of side effects	See separate list of contraindications	Initial: 10 bid Average: 20 Range: 10–50 Maximum: 60	See separate list of drug interactions

	Preparation (mg)	Mechanism of Action	Pharmaco-dynamics	Hemo-dynamics
Propranolol (Inderal)— Wyeth-Ayerst	10 20 40 60 80 90	Nonselective beta-adrenergic recep-tor blocker	Onset: 1–2 hr Peak: 2–4 hr Half-life: 2½–6 hr ISA: none MSA: 3+ Lipid solubility: high (4+) Metabolism: hepatic Excretion: hep-atic to renal	HR, CO, PRA, RPF, RBF, GFR, aldosterone reduced SVR and RVR increased MAP reduced Plasma volume increased
(Inderal LA)— Wyeth-Ayerst	60 80 120 160			
Timolol (Blocadren)— Merck	10 20	Nonselective beta-adrenergic re-ceptor blocking agent	Onset: ½–1 hr Peak: 1–2 hr Half-life: 3–4 hr ISA: none to minimal (1+) MSA: none Lipid solubility: low (2+) Metabolism: hepatic (80%) Excretion: renal (20%)	HR, CO, PRA, RPF, RBF, GFR, aldosterone reduced SVR, RVR increased MAP reduced Plasma volume increased
Alpha-beta–blocker Labetalol (Trandate)— Allen & Hanburys (Normodyne)— Schering-Plough	100 200 300 Also intra venous (5 mg/mL)	Competitive antag-onist at both alpha and beta receptors Oral: Alpha/beta ratio is 1:3 IV: Alpha/beta ratio is 1:7 Beta₂ agonist: Beta₁ and beta₂ antagonist; alpha₁ blocker; nonselective	Onset: 1 hr Peak: 2–4 hr Half-life: 6–8 hr ISA: none to 1+ MSA: 1+ Lipid solubility: low (1+) Metabolism: hepatic (40%) Excretion: renal (60%)	HR, CO, PRA reduced RPF, RBF, GFR unchanged to reduced SVR and RVR unchanged to slightly reduced MAP reduced Plasma volume increased or unchanged
Carvedilol (Coreg)— SmithKline Beecham	3.125 6.25 12.5 25	Nonselective beta-adrenergic blocker with alpha₁ blocking activity	Onset: ½ hr Absorption:80%, first pass in liver 23% Peak: 1–2 hr Half-life: 7–10 hr	Similar to labetalol, also mild calcium channel blocker, antioxidant and antiproliferative actions

Adverse Effects	Contraindications	Daily Dosage (mg)	Drug Interactions
See separate list of side effects	See separate list of contraindications	Initial: 40 Average: 80 bid Range: 10–640 Maximum: 640	See separate list of drug interactions
See separate list of adverse effects	See separate list of contraindications	Initial: 10 Average: 20 Range: 10–60 Maximum: 60	See separate list of drug interactions
See separate list of adverse effects	See separate list of contraindications	Initial: 100 bid Average: 200–400 bid Range: 400–800 Maximum: 2400	See separate list of drug interactions
Dizziness (6.2%) Fatigue (4.3%)	NYHA Class IV Asthma 2° or 3° AVB Bradycardia Cardiogenic shock Hepatic disease	Initial: 6.25 bid Average: 12.5 bid Maximum: 25 bid Take with food	Catecholamine- depleting agents Clonidine Digoxin Rifampin Diltiazem

	Preparation (mg)	Mechanism of Action	Pharmaco-dynamics	Hemo-dynamics
Carvedilol (continued)			ISA: none MSA: ? Lipid solubility: high Metabolism: hepatic (98%), P-450 enzymes Excretion: renal (2%)	
Bisoprolol (Zebeta)-Lederle	5 10	Beta, cardio-selective adreno-receptor blocking agent. Specificity lost with higher doses	Onset: 1 hr Peak: 2–4 hr ISA: none MSA: minimal to none Lipid solubility: low Metabolism: 50% hepatic 50% renal Excretions: 50% renal 50% nonrenal	HR, CO, PRA, RBF reduced MAP reduced SVR, RVP increased

*Consult the *Physicians' Desk Reference* for full prescribing information.

Adverse Effects	Contraindications	Daily Dosage (mg)	Drug Interactions
	Hypersensitivity to drug		Verapamil
			Insulin
			Oral hypoglycemics
			Cimetidine
See separate list of side effects	See separate list of contraindications	Initial: 5 Average: 10 Maximum: 20	See separate list of drug interactions

Direct Vasodilators

The direct vasodilators have a potent relaxation effect on the vascular smooth muscle of arteries, reducing SVR. The hemodynamics of the vasodilators are similar, but adverse effects differ. Because of increased PRA, CO, plasma volume, and reflex tachycardia, direct vasodilators require the concomitant use of either beta-blockers or central alpha-agonists and diuretics. The direct vasodilators hydralazine and minoxidil therefore should *not* be used alone (as monotherapy) to treat chronic hypertension. Minoxidil is much more potent than hydralazine. See Highlights next page.

Direct Vasodilators Highlights*

	Preparation	Mechanism of Action	Pharmacodynamics	Hemo-dynamics	Adverse Effects	Contra-indications	Daily Dosage	Drug Interactions
Hydralazine (Apresoline)— Novartis	10 mg 25 mg 50 mg 100 mg 20 mg/mL IV	Peripheral vasodilator that acts by direct relaxation on the vascular smooth muscles	Rapid absorption Duration: 6 hr Onset: 20–30 min (IV), 1 hr (oral) Peak: 2–4 hr Excretion: renal Metabolism: liver	Peripheral vasodilation SVR, PVR reduced HR, CO increased PRA increased GFR increased RBF, RPF increased	Postural hypo-tension Headaches Reflex tachy-cardia Nausea Palpitations Fatigue Fluid retention Lupus syndrome Nasal congestion	Aortic aneurysm Coronary artery disease Mitral valve or rheumatic heart disease	Initial: 10 mg qid Range: 40–400 mg Usual dose: 100–200 mg bid schedule	Diazoxide: severe hypotension Digoxin: decreased digoxin effect with IV hydra-lazine Beta-adrenergic blockers: en-hanced hydra-lazine effect
Minoxidil (Loniten)— Pharmacia & Upjohn	2.5 mg 5 mg 10 mg	Direct relaxation of arterial smooth muscle. Reduces SVR and PVR (little effect on venous smooth muscle)	Duration: 12 hr Onset: 1 hr Peak: 4–8 hr Excretion: renal Metabolism: liver	SVR, PVR reduced Reflex tachy-cardia HR, CO in-creased PRA, NE, Ang-II, aldos-terone in-creased RPF, RBF, GFR increased	Hypertrichosis Fluid retention and weight gain Precipitation of angina Cardiac tamponade ECG changes Reflex tachy-cardia	CHF Pheochromo-cytoma	Initial: 5 mg single dose Range: 10–40 mg bid schedule	Guanethidine: severe ortho-static hypo-tension

*Consult the *Physicians' Desk Reference* for full prescribing information.

Alpha$_1$-Blockers[103]

The alpha$_1$-blockers (indirect vasodilators) prazosin, doxazosin, and terazosin block the peripheral postsynaptic alpha$_1$-adrenergic receptor and reduce SVR but usually do not cause reflex tachycardia. CO is preserved or increased, and plasma volume is usually unchanged. These favorable hemodynamic changes reverse the abnormalities in essential hypertension and preserve organ perfusion.

Monotherapy with modest sodium restriction is effective in 50% to 60% of patients with mild hypertension. Concomitant use of diuretics is *not* necessarily required.

The alpha$_1$-blockers have no adverse effects on serum lipids and other CHD risk factors.

Side effects are infrequent and minor. First-dose syncope and hypotension are rare (less than 1%) and have been overemphasized. They are more likely to occur in patients who are volume depleted, are on diuretics, or are elderly.

Initiation at a low dose (1 mg hs) and slow titration to 10 mg/day improve compliance and minimize adverse effects while maximizing efficacy as initial monotherapy.

Alpha₁-Blockers Highlights*

	Preparation (mg)	Mechanism of Action	Pharmacodynamics
Doxazosin (Cardura)— Pfizer	1 2 4 8	Selective blockade of alpha₁ receptor. Antagonizes pressor effects of phenylephrine and NE	Duration: 24 hr Onset: 1 hr Peak: 2–6 hr Metabolism: liver Excretion: urinary and fecal
Prazosin (Minipress)— Pfizer	1 2 5 10	Vasodilator effect is related to blockade of peripheral post-synaptic alpha adrenoreceptors	Duration: 8–12 hr Onset: 1 hr Peak: 2–3 hr Metabolism: liver Excretion: biliary, feces
Terazosin (Hytrin)—Abbott	1 2 5 10	Postsynaptic alpha₁ blockade	Duration: 18–24 hr Onset: 1 hr Peak: 1–2 hr Metabolism: liver Excretion: biliary, feces

*Consult the *Physicians' Desk Reference* for full prescribing information.

Hemo-dynamics	Adverse Effects	Contra-indications	Daily Dosage (mg)	Drug Interactions
HR unchanged or increased CO unchanged SVR reduced Venous capacitance increased PRA unchanged RBF, RPF, GFR increased or unchanged PWP reduced or unchanged	Syncope (rare) Dizziness Increased sweating Fatigue Palpitations Edema	Hypersensitivity to quinazolines	Initial: 1 hs Maximum: 16 Average: 4–6	None
HR and CO unchanged or increased SVR reduced Venous capacitance increased PRA unchanged RPF, RBF, GFR unchanged or slightly increased PWP reduced or unchanged	Syncope with first dose (rare, <1%) Postural hypotension (uncommon) Palpitations Dizziness Weakness Headache	None	Initial: 1 bid with first dose at bedtime Maintenance: 5–15 in divided doses (bid) Maximum: 40	Beta-adrenergic blockers: increased hypotensive effect of the first dose Indomethacin: decreased hypotensive effect
See Prazosin	Syncope Postural hypotension Headache Tachycardia Asthenia Edema Dry mouth Nasal congestion Dizziness	None	Initial: 1 Average: 1–5 Maximum: 40; may require bid dosing	See Prazosin

Angiotensin-Converting Enzyme Inhibitors[103,104]

These agents inhibit the conversion of angiotensin I to angiotensin II, thus interrupting the renin-angiotensin-aldosterone system. Plasma renin activity is increased; angiotensin II and aldosterone levels are decreased. The net antihypertensive mechanism appears to be a decrease in fluid volume and vasodilation. ACE inhibitors may be used alone or in combination with other antihypertensive agents that enhance the effect. The agents may also affect the kinin-bradykinin and prostaglandin systems.

ACE inhibitors are most effective in high-renin and normal-renin hypertension and less effective in low-renin hypertension. Side effects are minor and infrequent, and most patients tolerate these agents well. Cough occurs in 10% to 15% of patients and is more common in women. ACE inhibitors are useful as initial therapy and as monotherapy. They are less effective in African-Americans and the elderly compared with whites and younger patients.

ACE inhibitors may also have a favorable effect in preserving renal function in both nondiabetic and diabetic hypertensives and reducing proteinuria and IGCP.

A triphasic BP response occurs with high renin levels:
1. Initial abrupt fall (occasionally to hypotensive levels) for several hours.
2. Return of BP but to below pretreatment levels.
3. Chronic gradual reduction of blood pressure over several days, but not as low as with initial therapy. Maximum effect at 2 to 4 weeks is predicted by initial response.

Patients with normal or low renin levels have a more prolonged and gradual decrease in BP. Volume depletion or concurrent antihypertensive therapy exaggerates the response.

There is no pseudotolerance, and dose can be reduced with time.

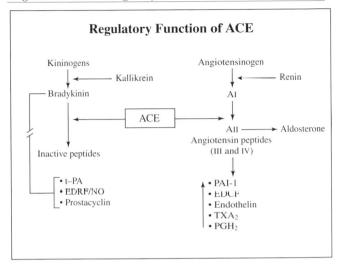

Regulatory Function of ACE

Adapted from Kang PM, Landau AJ, Eberhardt RT, Frishman WH. Angiotensin II receptor antagonists: A new approach to blockade of the renin-angiotensin system. Am Heart J. 1994;127:1388–1401.

ACE is the key enzyme in the RAAS and kinin system. ACE is found primarily in tissues such as the endothelium and blood vessels, where it stems from local synthesis secondary to gene expression. The adverse effects of ACE are related to its conversion of angiotensin I to angiotensin II and its degradation of bradykinin. In addition to causing vasoconstriction, increased angiotensin II levels, and an increase in PAI-1, EDCF and endothelin promote vascular smooth muscle growth and migration, matrix synthesis, platelet aggregation, and thrombosis. Degradation of bradykinin inhibits its vasodepressor, antiproliferative, and fibrinolytic effects due to decreases in endothelium-derived relaxing factor (EDRF)/NO, prostacyclin, and t-PA. The processes mediated by angiotensin II and bradykinin occur primarily at the tissue level and are implicated in a number of cardiovascular conditions, including hypertension, ischemia, atherosclerosis, vascular hypertrophy, and restenosis after vascular injury.

Consequences of Increased Vascular (Tissue) ACE

- ↑All production
  - Vasoconstriction
  - Growth factor release (e.g., PDGF)
  - Proto-oncogene activation
  - ↑ superoxide anion formation
  - Promotes thrombosis (e.g., ↑ PAI-1 via AIV)

- ↓ bradykinin production
  - ↓ NO and ↓ PGI_2 release
  - ↓ VSMC relaxation
  - Mediates inflammation (WBCs) and
    ↑ vascular permeability
  - ↓ fibrinolysis via ↓ t-PA

Adapted from Johnston CI. Renin-angiotensin system: A dual tissue and hormonal system for cardiovascular control. J Hypertens. 1992;10(Suppl 7):S13–S26.

Increased vascular ACE expression increases production of angiotensin II, which causes vasoconstriction, release of growth factors, and activation of proto-oncogenes that stimulate growth of vascular smooth muscle cells, and it enhances formation of superoxide anion, which promotes production of oxidized LDL cholesterol and atherosclerotic plaque formation. The vasoconstrictor effect of angiotensin II is mediated in large part by the sympathetic nervous system, which may explain the reduction in sympathetic tone that accompanies ACE inhibition. Increased vascular tissue ACE expression decreases bradykinin, thereby inhibiting its vasorelaxant and antiproliferative actions and increasing vascular permeability.

ACE Inhibitors Highlights*

	Preparation (mg)	Mechanism of Action	Pharmacodynamics
Benazepril (Lotensin)— Novartis	5 10 20 40	ACE Inhibitor	Onset: 1 hr Peak: 2–4 hr Plasma half-life: 10–11 hr Metabolism: hepatic, rena Excretion: renal Absorption: unaffected by food
Captopril (Capoten)— Bristol-Myers– Squibb	12.5 25 50 100	A specific inhibitor of angiotensin-converting enzyme; interrupts the renin-angiotensin system and formulation of angiotensin II	Onset: 1–2 hr Peak: 4 hr Plasma half-life: 8–12 hr (increases with dose) Metabolism: liver (15%) Excretion: renal (85%—unchanged 50% metabolites 35%) Absorption: reduced by food
Enalapril (Vasotec)— Merck	5 10 20	ACE Inhibitor	Onset: 1 hr Peak: 3–4 hr Plasma half-life: 12–24 hr Metabolism: liver Excretion: renal (40%) Absorption: unaffected by food

Hemo-dynamics	Adverse Effects	Contra-indications	Daily Dosage (mg)	Drug Interactions
Exercise response preserved	Headache	Similar to lisinopril	Initial: 10	Lithium
Angiotensin II and aldo-sterone reduced	Dizziness Fatigue		Average: 10–40	K⁺ supplements K⁺- sparing diuretics: risk of hyperkalemia
PRA and angio-tensin I increased	Cough Nausea Angioedema (rare)		Maximum: 80 Interval: qd	
GFR, RPF, RBF unchanged or increased				
RVR reduced				
HR unchanged or rarely increased				
SVR reduced				
MAP reduced				
See Benazepril	Taste distur-bances	Renal impair-ment	Initial: 25 bid or tid	Cimetidine: severe neuro-pathies in pa-tients with renal impairment
	Cutaneous rash Proteinuria Leukopenia Renal insuf-ficiency Cough Angioedema (rare)	Renal artery stenosis (caution) Connective tissue disease (caution)	Average: 100–150 Range: 75–450 Maximum: 450 Intervals: bid or tid Lower doses now recom-mended	Indomethacin: decreases hypo-tensive effect Spironolactone and triamterene: hyperkalemia (monitor K⁺ concentration) Lithium: Increased lithium levels K⁺ supplements, K⁺ sparing diu-retics (combina-tion, i.e., Dya-zide, Maxzide): risk of hyper-kalemia
See Benazepril	Less rash and loss of taste than with captopril Other side effects are similar	Renal impair-ment Renal artery stenosis (caution) Connective tis-sue disease (caution)	Initial: 5 Average: 20 Range: 10–140 Maximum: 40 Intervals: qid or bid	See Captopril

	Preparation (mg)	Mechanism of Action	Pharmacodynamics
Fosinopril (Monopril)— Bristol-Myers Squibb	10 20 40	ACE inhibitor	Onset: 1 hr Peak: 2–6 hr Plasma half-life: 12 hr Metabolism: hepatic, renal Excretion: renal, feces Absorption: unaffected by food
Quinapril (Accupril)— Parke-Davis	5 10 20 40	ACE inhibitor	Onset: 1 hr Peak: 1–2 hr Plasma half-life: 25 hr Metabolism: hepatic Excretion: renal (96%) Absorption: 60% decreased by food
Lisinopril (Prinivil)—Merck (Zestril)— Zeneca	5 10 20	ACE inhibitor	Onset: 1 hr Peak 6 hr Plasma half-life: 12–24 hr Metabolism: none Excretion: renal (100%) Absorption: unaffected by food
Ramipril (Altace)— Hoechst Marion Roussel	1.25 2.5 5 10	ACE inhibitor	Onset: 1 hr Peak: 3–6 hr Plasma half-life: 13–17 hr Metabolism: liver Excretion: renal (60%), hepatic (feces) (40%) Absorption: reduced by food
Moexipril (Univasc)— Schwarz	7.5 15	ACE inhibitor	Onset: 1 hr Peak: 1 ½ hr Plasma half-life: 12–14 hr Metabolism: liver Excretion: bile and urine Absorption: reduced by food
Trandolapril (Mavik)— Knoll	1 2 4	ACE inhibitor	Onset: 1 hr Peak: 4–10 hr Plasma half-life: 6–10 hr Metabolism: hepatic Excretion: urine, feces, bile
Perindopril (Aceon)— Rhone-Poulenc Rorer	2 mg 4 mg 8 mg	ACE inhibitor	Onset: 1 hour Peak: 3–7 hours Plasma half-life:3–10 hr Metabolism: Liver Excretion: Renal Absorption: Unaffected by food

*Consult the *Physicians' Desk Reference* for full prescribing information.
†Rare

Hemo-dynamics	Adverse Effects	Contra-indications	Daily Dosage (mg)	Drug Interactions
See Benazepril	Headache Dizziness Fatigue Cough Nausea Diarrhea Angioedema[†]	Similar to lisinopril	Initial: 10 Average: 20–40 Maximum: 80 Interval: qd	See above Digoxin: may cause false low digoxin levels
See Benazepril	Headache Fatigue Nausea Dizziness Cough Angioedema[†]	Hypersensitiv-ity to drug	Initial: 10 Average: 20–40 Maximum: 80 Interval: bid	See Captopril
See Benazepril	Dizziness Headache Fatigue Diarrhea Cough Interval: qd Angioedema[†] Hypotension[†] Neutropenia[†]	Hypersensitiv-ity to drug Renal impair-ment Renal artery stenosis (caution) Connective tis-sue disease (caution)	Initial: 5–10 monother-apy Average: 20–40 Maximum: 80 Interval: qd	Diuretics: hypotension Indomethacin renal insuffi-ciency K+-sparing agents and K+ supple-ments: increased risk of hyper-kalemia
See Benazepril	Headache Dizziness Fatigue Cough Nausea Angioedema[†]	Hypersensitiv-ity to drug	Initial: 2.5 Average: 2.5–20 Maximum: 20 Interval: qd	Benazepril
	As above	As above	Initial: 7.5 Maximum: 30 Interval:qd	As above
See Benazepril	Cough Dizziness Diarrhea Headache Fatigue	As above	Initial: 1–2 Average: 2–4 Maximum: 4 Interval: qd or bid	As above
See Benazepril	Dizziness Headache Asthenia Rhinitis Dyspepsia Proteinuria Palpitations	History of angio-edema related to previous ACE inhibitor Pregnancy Renal impair-ment (caution) Renal artery stenosis (caution)	Initial: 4 mg qd Average: 4–8 mg Maximum: 16 mg Intervals: qd or bid	Diuretic: hypo-tension K+ sparing agents and K+ supple-ments may increase risk of hyperkalemia Gentamicin use with caution

Calcium Channel Blockers[147]

Calcium channel blockers inhibit the influx of calcium ions through slow channels in vascular smooth muscle tissue and cause relaxation of the arterioles of the body. These agents are useful in the treatment of all degrees of hypertension (mild, moderate, or severe).

1. The higher the BP, the greater the therapeutic reduction in BP.
2. Low-renin hypertensive patients (volume-dependent patients) have the best response (75% to 80% response rate as monotherapy), but most patients respond well.
3. African-Americans and elderly patients also respond well (75% to 80% with monotherapy).
4. Mild edema in the absence of weight gain may be seen with long-term use. Diuretic and natriuretic effects occur. ACEI will counteract this edema.
5. Antihypertensive effect is enhanced by most other antihypertensive agents.
6. The effect on lipids is neutral or favorable. No adverse effect is seen on K^+, Mg^{2+}, glucose, uric acid, etc.
7. There is a low adverse effect profile.
8. Calcium channel blockers inhibit development of atherosclerosis in animal and human coronary arteries and cause regression of early atherosclerotic lesions.
9. Calcium channel blockers preserve renal function.
10. LVH is reduced.
11. Calcium channel blockers are very effective as monotherapy.
12. Calcium channel blockers have been shown to reduce incidence of dementia (cognitive function improves with reduction in blood pressure). (Forette F, Seux ML, Staessen JA, et al. Prevention of dementia in randomised double-blind placebo-controlled Systolic Hypertension in Europe (Syst-Eur) trial. Lancet 1998;352:1347–1351.)
13. Amlodipine increases nitric oxide levels, which improves endothelial function, decreases alpha tumor necrosis factor (TNF), decreases membrane width and smooth muscle cell proliferation, is a potent antioxidant, and reduces PDGF.

Calcium Channel Blockers Highlights

	Preparation	Mechanism of Action	Pharmacodynamics
Amlodipine	2.5 mg	Coronary and	Absorption: 100% unaltered by food
(Norvasc)—Pfizer	5 mg	vascular smooth	Bioavailability:
	10 mg	muscle vasodilation	64%–90%
			Onset: 6 hrs
			Peak: 6–12 hrs
			Half-life: 30–50 hrs
			Protein binding: 93%
			Metabolism: hepatic: 90%
			Excretion: urine (60%): metabolites
			No alteration with renal insufficiency
Diltiazem SR	60 mg	Selective relaxa-	Absorption: well
(Cardizem SR,	90 mg	tion of smooth	absorbed >90%
Cardizem CD)—	120 mg	muscle	Bioavailability:
Hoechst	120 mg		45%–67% (first
Marion	180 mg		pass-hepatic)
Roussel	240 mg		Onset: 1 hr
	300 mg		Peak: 3 hrs
			Half-life: 4 hrs
			Protein binding: 80%
(Tiazac)—	120 mg	Relaxation of	Metabolism: hepatic
Forest/UAD	180 mg	smooth muscle	(60% fecal excretion)
	240 mg		Excretion: renal (35%)
	300 mg		Plasma levels: 40–
	360 mg		200 ng/mL
(Dilacor XR)—	180 mg	Relaxation of	
Rhone Poulenc	240 mg	smooth muscle	
Rorer	360 mg		
(Tiamate)—	180 mg	Relaxation of	
Hoechst Marion	240 mg	smooth muscle	
Roussel	360 mg		
Isradipine	2.5 mg	Selective relaxation	Absorption:
(DynaCirc,	5 mg	of smooth muscle	90%–95%
DynaCirc SR†)—	10 mg	in systemic vascu-	Bioavailability:
Novartis		lature. Mild	15%–24%
		diuretic activity	Onset of action: 20 min
			Peak: 2–3 hr
			Food increases time to peak by 1 hr

Hemo-dynamics	Adverse Effects	Contra-indications	Daily Dosage (mg)	Drug Interactions
SVR reduced HR unchanged CO unchanged or increased RBF, RPF, GFR preserved, increased No effect on sinotrial (SA) or AV node Coronary vasodilation Afterload reduction Dilates coronary and peripheral arteries	Dizziness Palpitations Flushing Edema	Hypersensitivity to drug	Initial: 5 Average: 5 Maximum: 10 Interval: qd Long T 1/2 - intrinsic High trough to peak ratio	None yet established
Depresses SA and AV nodal function Negative inotropic effect Reduces HR Reduces SVR Increases MVO^2 CO unchanged	Headache AV block disorders and sinus arrest Dizziness Pedal edema Bradycardia Electrocardiographic abnormalities Asthenia Constipation Dyspepsia Nausea Palpitations	Sick sinus syndrome, AV block (2nd-degree, 3rd-degree), severe CHF, digitalis toxicity Acute MI and pulmonary congestion Additive effects with beta blockers and digoxin	Average: 240–360 Range: 120–360 Maximum: 360 Interval: bid or tid Initial: 120–240 Average: 180–360 Maximum: 540 Interval: once daily	Beta-adrenergic blockers: cardiac failure (additive effects on contractility and blockade of compensating reflexes) AV conduction disturbances and sinus bradycardia (additive)
Vasodilation with increased coronary, cerebral, and skeletal muscle blood flow SVR reduced HR increased CO increased	Headache Dizziness Edema Palpitations Fatigue Flushing	Hypersensitivity to drug	Initial: 2.5 bid Average: 5–10 in divided doses Maximum: 20	

	Preparation	Mechanism of Action	Pharmacodynamics
Isradipine (*continued*)			Half-life: biphasic; early: 1½–2 hr terminal: 8 hr Protein binding: 95% Excretion: urine 60%–65%, feces 25%–30%
Nicardipine (Cardene)— Roche	20 mg 30 mg	Selective relaxation of vascular smooth muscle. More selective on	Absorption: >95% Bioavailability: 35% Onset: 30 min Peak: 1 hr
(Cardene SR)— Roche	45 mg 60 mg	smooth muscle than myocardium. Greater effect on cerebral and coronary vessels than peripheral vessels	Half-life: 8.6 hr Protein binding: 95% Metabolism: liver Excretion: urine 60%, feces 35% Plasma levels: 10–100 ng/mL
Nifedipine (Adalat CC)— Bayer	30 mg 60 mg extended-release tablets	Selective relaxation of vascular smooth muscle by reducing intracellular calcium concentration in	*Absorption: 90% Bioavailability: 43% Onset: 2 hr Plateau: 6 hr Half-life: 2 hr
(Procardia XL)— Pfizer	90 mg	coronary and systemic vasculature	Protein binding: 92%–98% Metabolism: liver—complete Excretion: renal (60%–80%) Plasma levels: 20–90 ng/mL

*Absorption of Adalat is altered with food, whereas Procardia XL is not.

Hemo-dynamics	Adverse Effects	Contra-indications	Daily Dosage (mg)	Drug Interactions
SVR reduced Reflex increase in HR MAP reduced RBF, RPF, GFR preserved CO unchanged or increased No effect on sinoatrial or AV nodal conduction Coronary artery vasodilation	Flushing Headache Pedal edema Asthenia Palpitations Dizziness Tachycardia	Advanced aortic stenosis Hypersensitivity to drug	Initial: 20 tid Average: 30 tid Maximum: 40 tid	Food: increases time to peak by 1 hr Cimetidine: increases nicardipine levels Cyclosporine: increases cyclosporine plasma levels Beta-blockers: CHF
SVR (peripheral arterial vasodilation) reduced PRA decreased MAP reduced RBF, RPF, GFR preserved CO increased or unchanged by reflex sympathetic activity and decreased SVR No effect on sinoatrial or AV nodal function Myocardial oxygen supply increased by increasing coronary artery blood flow and decreasing myocardial oxygen demand Smooth muscle relaxation (generalized)	Headache Dizziness Lightheadedness Tremor Nervousness Palpitations Leg cramps Fatigue Weakness Nausea Diarrhea Edema Flushing Orthostatic hypotension Tinnitus	Hypersensitivity to drug	Initial: 30 Average: 30 Range: 30–60 Maximum: 60 Interval: qd	Beta-adrenergic blockers: cardiac failure (additive effects on contractility and blockade of compensating reflexes) Digoxin: increased digoxin effect (rare) Hypoglycemics, sulfonylurea: decreased hypoglycemic effect with oral nifedipine (decreased glucose metabolism) Cimetidine: increased nifedipine plasma levels Food alters Adalat CC absorption.

	Preparation	Mechanism of Action	Pharmacodynamics
Nifedipine (Adalat CC)— Bayer (Procardia XL)— Pfizer	30 mg 60 mg 90 mg extended- release tablets	Selective relaxation of vascular smooth muscle by reducing intracellular cal- cium concentration	Absorption: 90% Bioavailability: 75% Onset: immediate First peak: 2.5–5 hr Second peak: 6–12 hr Half-life: 2 hr Protein binding: 92%–98% Metabolism: liver— complete Excretion: renal (60%–80%) Plasma levels: C_{max} is 36% greater avg con- centration 70% greater in sub- jects age >60 yr 6–120 ng/mL
Nisoldipine (Sular)— Zeneca	10 mg 20 mg 30 mg 40 mg	Inhibits calcium influx into vascular smooth muscle and cardiac muscle	Absorption: 87% Bioavailability: 5% Onset: 2 hr Peak: 6–12 hr Half-life: 7–12 hr Protein binding: 99% Metabolism: liver Excretion: urine (60%–80%)

Hemo-dynamics	Adverse Effects	Contra-indications	Daily Dosage (mg)	Drug Interactions
SVR reduced PRA decreased MAP reduced RBF, RPF, GFR preserved CO increased or unchanged by reflex sympathetic activity and decreased SVR No effect on sinoatrial or AV nodal function Smooth muscle relaxation (generalized)	Headache Dizziness Lightheadedness Tachycardia Tremor Nervousness Palpitations Leg cramps Fatigue Weakness Nausea Diarrhea Edema Flushing Orthostatic hypotension Tinnitus	Hypersensitivity to drug	Initial: 30 Average: 30 Range: 30–90 Maximum: 90 Interval: qd on empty stomach	Beta-adrenergic blockers: cardiac failure (additive effects on contractility and blockade of compensating-reflexes) Digoxin: increased digoxin effect (rare) Hypoglycemics, sulfonylurea: increased hypoglycemic effect with oral nifedipine (decreased glucose metabolism) Cimetidine: increased nifedipine plasma levels
Similar to nifedipine	Similar to nifedipine	Allergy	Average: 20 Range: 10–60 qd Maximum: 60	Cimetidine: increased plasma levels Quinidine: decreased bioavailability

	Preparation	Mechanism of Action	Pharmacodynamics
Verapamil (Calan SR)— Searle (Isoptin SR)— Knoll (Verelan)— Wyeth-Ayerst Verelan PM— (Schwarz)	Oral: 240 mg SR tab 120 mg 180 mg 200 mg 300 mg	Selective relaxation of smooth muscle by reducing intra-cellular calcium concentration in coronary and peri-pheral vasculature and inhibiting slow-channel Ca^{2+} transport	Absorption: 95% Bioavailability: 10%–20% (extensive hepatic first pass) Onset: 1 hr Peak: 2 hr Half-life: 3–6 hr (up to 9 hr with long-term therapy) Protein binding: 90% Metabolism: hepatic (85%) fecal (15%); accumu-lates in liver disease Excretion: renal (70%), biexponential elimina-tion (fast/slow) Plasma levels: 80–300 ng/mL
Covera HS)— Searle	180 mg 240 mg	See above. Unique delivery system designed for 4–5 hr delay to be taken hs for max. concentration in the A.M.	Absorption: 65% Bioavailability: 33%–65% Onset: 4–5 hr Peak: 11 hr Half-life: 14–16 hr Protein binding: 94% Metabolism: hepatic Excretion: renal (70%), fecal (16%)
Felodipine (Plendil)—Astra	5 mg 10 mg	Selective relaxation of vascular smooth muscle, more than on myocardium	Absorption: 95% Bioavailability: 20% Onset: 1/2-1 hr Peak: 2.5-5 hr Half-life: 11-16 hr Protein binding: 99% Metabolism: liver Excretion: urine 70% feces 10%

---

*Consult the *Physicians' Desk Reference* for full prescribing information.
†Not found in *Physicians' Desk Reference*.

Hemo-dynamics	Adverse Effects	Contra-indications	Daily Dosage (mg)	Drug Interactions
Sinoatrial and AV nodal function depressed reentrant pathways, ventricular response slowed SVR arterial reduced (no venous effect) MAP reduced—less pronounced CO reduced, negative inotropic action Mild bradycardia Myocardial oxygen supply increased by increasing coronary blood flow Myocardial oxygen demand reduced by decreasing HR and reducing afterload No adverse effect on pulmonary function Smooth muscle relaxation—generalized (vascular, gut, bronchial)	Constipation: most common Headache Vertigo, dizziness, light-headedness Weakness Nervousness Pruritus, flushing Gastric disturbances Hepatitis SGOT Alkaline phosphatase Orthostatic hypotension AV block AV dissociation Asystole Sinus arrest Pedal edema Pulmonary edema and CHF Paresthesias (cold, numbness) Hyperprolactinemia and galactorrhea	Sick sinus syndrome, second-degree or third-degree AV block, digitalis toxicity, cardiogenic shock	Average: 240 Range: 120–480 Maximum: 480 Interval: qd, bid Average: 240 Range: 180–480 Maximum: 480 Interval: qhs (swallow whole)	Beta-adrenergic blockers: cardiac failure (additive effects on contractility and blockade of compensating reflexes) Digoxin: increased digoxin toxicity (possibly decreased renal excretion) Hypoglycemics, sulfonylurea: increased hypoglycemic effect (increased glucose metabolism) Lithium: increased lithium levels Rifampin: reduced bioavailability of Calan Carbamazepine: increased carbamazepine concentrations Neuromuscular blocking agents: Calan may potentiate their effects
SRV reduced HR increased RBF, RPF, GFR preserved CO unchanged or increased No effect on SA or AV conduction Coronary artery vasodilation	Edema Headache Flushing Dizziness Asthenia Tachycardia Fatigue Extrasystoles Nausea Palpitations	Hypersensitivity to drug	Initial: 5 mg Average 5-10 mg Maximum: 20 mg Adjust every 2 weeks if necessary Take tablet whole	Cimetidine: increased felodipine levels Digoxin: increased digoxin levels Phenytoin, carbamazepine, phenobarbital: decreased felodipine levels

Angiotensin II Receptor Blockers (ARBs)

Ang-II receptor blockers are the newest class of antihypertensives. Like ACE inhibitors, these agents interfere with the renin-angiotensin-aldosterone system. ACE inhibitors block the conversion of A-I to Ang-II, whereas ARBs block the binding of Ang-II to one of its receptor sites, AT_1. It is thought that the actions of Ang-II are more effectively blocked by direct AT_1 receptor antagonism.

Ang-II receptor blockers have a more favorable safety and tolerability profile than ACE inhibitors. They do not cause the adverse effects, such as cough and angioedema, that are attributed to ACE inhibitor interactions with the bradykinin system.

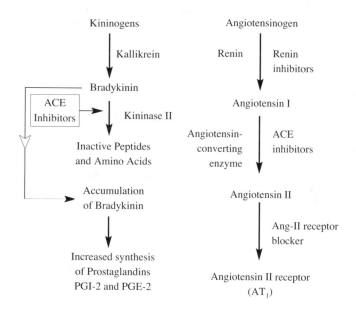

Interrupting the Renin System

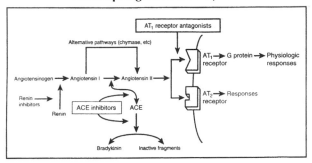

Site of angiotensin II type 1 (AT$_1$) receptor antagonists and angiotensin-converting enzyme (ACE) inhibitors in the renin-angiotensin-aldosterone system. (Adapted from Johnston CI: Angiotensin receptor antagonists: focus on losartan. Lancet 1995;346:1403-1407.)

Angiotensin II Receptors and the Effects of Blockade

Vascular AT$_1$ receptors
        Constantly expressed
        Mediate vasoconstriction
        Mediate angiotensin II arterial wall growth effects
Vascular AT$_2$ receptors
        Expressed only after injury (sustained hypertension
          might provoke expression)
        Mediate vasodilation
        Mediate antiproliferative actions
        Activate other factors (e.g., nitric oxide)
Potential double action of selective AT$_1$ blockers
        Directly block vasoconstrictor and growth actions of
          angiotensin II at AT$_1$ receptors
        Increase circulating angiotensin II levels
        Unblocked AT$_2$ receptors (if expressed), stimulated by
          increased angiotensin II activity, mediate vasodilation
          and growth inhibition
        Net effects: AT$_1$, blockade + AT$_2$ stimulation
        Unknown effect on other AT receptors.

AT1, angiotensin II type 1; AT2, angiotensin II type 2.
From Weber MA: Interrupting the renin-angiotensin system: The role of angiotensin-converting enzyme inhibitors and angiotensin II receptor antagonists in the treatment of hypertension. Am J Hypertens 1999;12:189S-194S.

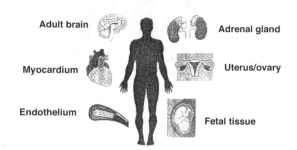

Adult brain

Adrenal gland

Myocardium

Uterus/ovary

Endothelium

Fetal tissue

Distribution of the AT2 receptor, which is ubiquitous in fetal tissue, and is present in high concentrations in adults only in the adrenal medulla, uterus, ovary, vascular endothelium, and distinct brain areas. (From Chung O, Unger T: Angiotensin II receptor blockade and end-organ protection. Am J Hypertens 1999;12:150S-156S, with permission.)

Examples of Genes That Can Be Regulated by Angiotensin II

Early genes/ proto-oncogenes
fos, myc, myb, jun, jun-B, egr-1

Growth factor genes
Transforming growth factor β_1, platelet-derived growth factor-A chain, fibroblast growth factor-2, insulin-like growth factor-1 receptor

Cell matrix factor genes
Fibronectin, collagen type 1-α_1, collagen type III-α_1, laminin-β_1, laminin-β_2,

Hypertrophic marker
Atrial natriuretic peptide, brain natriuretic peptide, skeletal muscle action-α_1,

Fibrinolytic system genes
Plasminogen activator inhibitor, types 1 and 2

Miscellaneous genes
Aldosterone synthase (CYP11B2), endothelial nitric oxide synthase

From Kurtz TW, Gardner DG: Transcription-modulating drugs: a new frontier in the treatment of essential hypertension. Hypertension 1998;32:380-386. December 1999-Vol. 12, No. 12, Part 3, with permission.

Pharmacologic Properties of Available ARB

Compound	Solubility in Water/Alcohol	Bioavailability (%)	Food Effect	Active Metabolite	Half-life (h)	Protein Binding (%)	Dosing (mg)
Irbesartan[8]	–/*	60-80	No	No	11-15	90	150-300 daily
Losartan[9] (EXP 3174)	+/+	33	Minimal	Yes	2 (6-9)	98.7 (99.8)	50-100 daily, twice daily
Valsartan[10]	*/+	25	40%-50% decrease	No	6	95	80-320 daily
Candesartan[11]	–/*	15	No	Yes	9	>99	8-32 daily, twice daily
Telmisartan[12]	–/NR	42-58	6%-20% decrease	No	24	99.5	40-80 daily
Eprosartan	-	13	Yes Minimal < 25%	No	5-9	98	400-600 daily

*Low solubility; NR, not reported.

From Zusman RM: Are there differences among angiotensin receptor blockers? Am J Hypertens 1999:12:231S-235S, with permission.

Ang-II Receptor Blockers (ARBs) Highlights*

Preparation	Mechanism of Action	Pharmaco-dynamics	Hemo-dynamics	Adverse Effects	Contra-indications	Daily Dosage	Drug Interactions
Candesartan cilexetil (Atacand)— Astra 4 mg 8 mg 16 mg 32 mg	Selective AT_1 angiotension II receptor antoagonist (see Irbesartan)	Onset: 0.5 hr Peak: 3–4 hr Plasma half-life: 9 hr Metabolism: hepatic and renal Excretion: urine and feces	(see Irbesartan)	Headache Dizziness Upper respiratory infections Pharyngitis Rhinitis	Pregnancy Hypersensitivity to drug	Initial: 16 mg qd Range: 8–32 mg Maximum: 32 mg qd	No significant interactions reported
Eprosartan (Teveten)— Unimed 400 mg 600 mg	ARB	Peak 1–2 hrs T 1/2 5–9 hrs Metabolism:none Excretion:bile Absorption:13%	Similar to other ARBs	Rare facial edema Similar to other ARBs	Pregnancy Hypersensitivity	400–800 mg	None
Irbesartan (Avapro)— Bristol Myers Squibb 75 mg 150 mg 300 mg	Blocks vasoconstrictor and aldosterone-secreting effects of angiotensin II by selectively binding to the AT_1 angiotensin II receptor.	Peak: 1.5–2 hr Plasma half-life: 11–15 hr Metabolism: biliary and renal Excretion: urine: 20% feces: 80% Absorption: (not affected by food) 60–80%	Exercise response preserved AII and PRA increased Aldosterone reduced No effect on bradykinin GFR, RPF, RBF unchanged MAP reduced HR unchanged	Diarrhea Dyspepsia/ heartburn Musculo-skeletal trauma Fatigue Upper respiratory infection	Hypersensitivity to drug Pregnancy	Initial: 150 mg qd Range: 150–300 mg Maximum: 300 mg qd	May be administered with other hypertensives. Hydro-chlorothiazide has shown additive . effect

Losartan (Cozaar)— Merck	25 and 50 mg	Blocks vasoconstrictor and aldosterone-secreting effects of Ang-II	Onset: 1 hr Peak: 3–4 hr (active metabolite) Plasma half-life: 6–9 hr (active metabolite) Metabolism: hepatic and renal Excretion: renal and biliary Absorption: food slows absorption	Exercise response preserved Ang-II and PRA increased Aldosterone reduced No effect on bradykinin GFR, RPF, RBF unchanged MAP reduced HR unchanged	Dizziness Asthenia/ fatigue Headache Cough	Pregnancy Hypersensitivity Caution with decreased liver function	Initial: 25– 50 mg Range: 25– 100 mg qd or bid Maximum: 100 mg qd or bid	May be administered with other hypertensives
Telmisartan (Micardis)— Boehringer Ingelheim	40 mg 80 mg	(see Irbesartan)	Peak: 0.5–1 hr Plasma half-life: 24 hr Metabolism: gut wall Excretion: feces (>97%) Absorption: slightly affected by food	(see Irbesartan)	Upper respiratory infection Back pain Sinusitis Diarrhea Pharyngitis	Pregnancy Nursing mothers Hypersensitivity to drug Caution with biliary obstruction and hepatic insufficiency	Initial: 40 mg qd Range: 20– 80 mg qd Maximum: 80 mg qd	Digoxin: ↑ peak plasma concentration

Continued on next page.

Ang-II Receptor Blockers (ARBs) Highlights (*Continued*)*

	Preparation	Mechanism of Action	Pharmaco-dynamics	Hemo-dynamics	Adverse Effects	Contra-indications	Daily Dosage	Drug Interactions
Valsartan (Diovan) Novartis	80 mg caps 160 mg caps	Blocks the vasocon-strictor and aldosterone secreting effects of AII by selectively blocking binding of AII to AT$_1$ receptor tissues.	Onset: 2 hr Peak: 2–4 hr Half-life: 6 hr Metabolism: liver and renal Absorption: 30–50% Excretion: urine 13%, feces 83%	Exercise response preserved AII and PRA increased Aldosterone reduced No effect on bradykinin GFR, RPF, RBF unchanged MAP reduced HR unchanged	Headache Dizziness Viral infections Fatigue Abdominal pain	Hypersensitive to drug Pregnancy Caution with elevated liver function tests	Initial: 80 mg qd Average: 80–160 mg qd Maximum: 320 mg qd Maximal BP reduction seen in 4 weeks	No significant interactions reported

*Consult the *Physicians' Desk Reference* for full prescribing information.

162

Selected Combination Antihypertensive Drugs

Beta-Adrenergic Blockers and Diuretics

Atenolol, 50 or 100 mg/chlorthalidone, 25 mg — Tenoretic

Bisoprolol fumarate, 2.5, 5, or 10 mg/hydrochlorothiazide, 6.25 mg — Ziac

Metoprolol tartrate, 50 or 100 mg/ hydrochlorothiazide, 25 or 50 mg — Lopressor HCT

Nadolol, 40 or 80 mg/bendroflumethiazide, 5 mg — Corzide

Propranolol hydrochloride, 40 or 80 mg/hydro-chlorothiazide, 25 mg — Inderide

Propranolol hydrochloride (extended release), 80, 120, or 160 mg/hydrochlorothiazide, 50 mg — Inderide LA

Timolol maleate, 10 mg/hydrochlorothiazide, 25 mg — Timolide

ACE Inhibitors and Diuretics

Benazepril hydrochloride, 5, 10, or 20 mg/ hydrochlorothiazide, 6.25, 12.5, or 25 mg — Lotensin HCT

Captopril, 25 or 50 mg/hydrochlorothiazide, 15 or 25 mg — Capozide

Enalapril maleate, 5 or 10 mg/hydrochlorothiazide, 12.5 or 25 mg — Vaseretic

Lisinopril, 10 or 20 mg/hydrochlorothiazide, 12.5 or 25 mg — Prinzide, Zestoretic

Angiotensin II Receptor Blockers and Diuretics

Valsartan, 80 or 160 mg/hydrochlorothiazide, 12.5 mg — Diovan HCT

Losartan potassium, 50 mg/hydrochlorothiazide, 12.5 mg — Hyzaar

Calcium Antagonists and ACE Inhibitors

Amlodipine besylate, 2.5 or 5 mg/benazepril hydrochloride, 10 or 20 mg — Lotrel

Diltiazem hydrochloride, 180 mg/enalapril maleate, 5 mg — Teczem

Verapamil hydrochloride (extended release), 180 or 240 mg/trandolapril, 1, 2, or 4 mg — Tarka

Felodipine, 5 mg/enalapril maleate, 5 mg — Lexxel

Other Combinations

Triamterene, 37.5, 50, or 75 mg/hydrochlorothiazide, 25 or 50 mg — Dyazide, Maxide

Spironolactone, 25 or 50 mg/hydrochlorothiazide, 25 or 50 mg — Aldactazide

Amiloride hydrochloride, 5 mg/hydrochlorothiazide, 50 mg — Moduretic

Guanethidine monosulfate, 10 mg/hydrochlorothiazide, 25 mg — Esimil

Hydralazine hydrochloride, 25, 50, or 100 mg/hydro-chlorothiazide, 25 or 50 mg — Apresazide

Methyldopa, 250 or 500 mg/hydrochlorothiazide, 15, 25, 30, or 50 mg — Aldoril

Reserpine, 0.125 mg/hydrochlorothiazide, 25 or 50 mg — Hydropres

Reserpine, 0.10 mg/hydralazine hydrochloride, 25 mg/ hydrochlorothiazide, 15 mg — Ser-Ap-Es

Clonidine hydrochloride, 0.1, 0.2, or 0.3 mg/chlor-thalidone, 15 mg — Combipres

Methyldopa, 250 mg/chlorothiazide, 150 or 250 mg — Aldochlor

Reserpine, 0.125 or 0.25 mg/chlorthalidone, 25 or 50 mg — Demi-Regroton

Reserpine, 0.125 or 0.25 mg/chlorothiazide, 250 or 500 mg — Diupres

Prazosin hydrochloride, 1, 2, or 5 mg/polythiazide, 0.5 mg — Minizide

Hypertension Drug Selection: *Summary*

- Calcium channel blockers (CCBs), angiotensin receptor blockers (ARBs), and angiotensin-converting enzyme inhibitors (ACEIs) have the best overall profile based on the eight parameters in the subsets of approach to hypertension.
- Combination therapy (low dose) with CCBs, ACEIs, and ARBs may provide synergistic antihypertensive effects, reduce side effects, and improve surrogate endpoints as well as target organ damage.
- Clinical trials in hypertension with CCBs reduce CHD, MI, and CVA equal to or better than diuretics and beta-blockers. ACEIs are equal to diuretics and beta blockers in reducing cardiovascular morbidity and mortality in recent clinical trials.
- Clinical trials in hypertension with ACEIs, ARBs, central alpha agonists, and alpha blockers are in progress to prove reduction in target organ damage. However, clinical trials in CHF show benefit with ACEIs and ARBs, and clinical trials in MI show benefit with ACEIs.
- Diuretics should be second-line or third-line therapy and never exceed 25 mg/day of HCTZ or its equivalent. Their impact on CHD and MI is suboptimal, whereas CVA is reduced, as expected.
- Beta-blockers as monotherapy do not reduce CHD or MI in the elderly population, and their efficacy in younger populations is questionable. Beta-blockers do reduce CVA and are effective in reducing morbidity after an acute MI.
- Central alpha-agonists and alpha-blockers are effective as monotherapy or as add-on therapy with metabolic profiles but may be limited due to side effects, unless kept at very low doses.
- In patients with diabetes mellitus and hypertension, recent clinical trials indicate that CCBs and ACEIs are superior to diuretics and beta-blockers in reducing cardiovascular and cerebrovascular morbidity and mortality.

New Antihypertensive Drug Classes

1. Renin inhibitors
2. Vasopressin antagonists
3. Neuropeptidase inhibitors
4. Serotonin receptor antagonists (ketanserin)
5. Dopamine receptor antagonists (fenoldopam)
6. Prostaglandin analogs (PGI_2-iloprost)
7. Lipoxygenase inhibitors (phenidone)
8. Cicletanine
9. Potassium channel activators (BRL-34915)
10. Sodium channel blockers (6-iodoamiloride)
11. Endothelin antagonists

Conclusions

1. The treatment of mild hypertension (DBP <110 mm Hg) with certain antihypertensive agents may induce metabolic or structural changes and adversely affect other risk factors that *partially or completely* negate the beneficial effects of lowering BP because of increases in CHD risk or risk factors for other end-organ damage.

2. Diuretic agents (except spironolactone and indapamide), beta-blockers without ISA, reserpine, and methyldopa have adverse effects on the hypertensive-atherosclerotic syndrome and other risk factors for end organ damage. These agents also have significant clinical side effects with a corresponding poor quality of life.

3. The only antihypertensive agents available to date that do not adversely affect serum lipids are calcium channel blockers, alpha$_1$-blockers, central alpha-agonists (except methyldopa), ACE inhibitors, indapamide, and Ang-II receptor blockers. All of these agents are effective as initial monotherapy in about 50% to 60% or more of patients with mild hypertension. All are well tolerated (in >90% of patients) if dosed appropriately (start low, go slow) and have a low side-effect profile. Combination therapy is 90% to 95% effective.

4. Diuretic agents in high doses (50 to 100 mg of HCTZ daily or an equivalent diuretic) may induce hypokalemia, hypomagnes-

emia, or other electrolyte and acid-base abnormalities that increase the incidence of sudden death in predisposed patients secondary to cardiac arrhythmias. Predisposing factors include exercise, the presence of LVH, abnormal ECGs, silent or clinical ischemia, acute stress, or digitalis treatment. Avoid these high doses.

5. The use of lower doses of diuretics (HCTZ 12.5 to 25 mg/day) is effective for the treatment of hypertension and may have fewer adverse effects. A dose of 25 mg/day achieves 95% of the antihypertensive effect and 12.5 mg achieves 80% of the antihypertensive effect.[108] Indapamide is a preferred diuretic.

6. The selection of nonpharmacologic therapy or antihypertensive drugs that have a neutral or favorable effect on serum lipids, glucose, electrolytes, and other risk factors and improve endothelial function may reduce the risk of CHD and other end-organ damage in patients with hypertension. *Optimal* treatment aims to reduce *all* risk factors, thereby reducing *all* end-organ damage.

7. Selection of drug therapy should be individualized and based on the subsets of hypertension approach and reversing the components of the hypertension-atherosclerotic syndrome.

Subset Selection of Antihypertensive Therapy

1. Pathophysiology and vascular biology
2. Hemodynamics
3. End-organ damage and risk factor reduction
4. Concomitant medical diseases or problems
5. Demographic selection
6. Adverse effects and quality of life with therapy
7. Compliance
8. Total health care cost

References

1. Levy RI. Lipid regulation: A new era in the prevention of coronary heart disease. Am Heart J. 1985;110:1099–1100.

2. Collins JG. Physician visits: Volume and interval since last visit, United States, 1980. U.S. Department of Health and Human Services (PHS) publication 83–1572, Series 10, No. 144, 1983.

3. Kannel WB. Some lessons in cardiovascular epidemiology from Framingham. Am J Cardiol. 1976;37:269–282.

4. Houston MC. Hypertension strategies for therapeutic intervention and prevention of end-organ damage. Primary Care Clin North Am. 1991; 18:713–753.

5. Houston MC. New insights and approaches to reduce end organ damage in the treatment of hypertension: Subsets of hypertension approach. Am Heart J. 1992;123:1337–1367.

6. The Fifth Report of the Joint National Committee on Detection, Evaluation, and Treatment of High Blood Pressure (JNC V). Arch Intern Med. 1993;153:154–183.

7. Kirkendall WM, Feinleib M, Freis ED, Mark AL. Recommendations for human blood pressure determination by sphygmomanometers: Subcommittee of the AHA Postgraduate Education Committee. Circulation. 1980;62:1146A–1155A.

8. Final Report of the Subcommittee on Nonpharmacological Therapy of the 1984 Joint National Committee on Detection, Evaluation, and Treatment of High Blood Pressure: Nonpharmacological approaches to the control of high blood pressure. Hypertension. 1986;8:444–467.

9. Houston MC. New insights and new approaches for the treatment of essential hypertension: Selections of therapy based on coronary heart disease risk factor analysis, hemodynamic profiles, quality of life, and subsets of hypertension. Am Heart J. 1989;117:911–951.

10. Hollifield JW, Slaton P. Demographic approach to initiation of antihypertensive therapy: Treatment strategies in hypertension. Miami: Symposium Specialists, Inc. 1981:51–58.

11. Woods JW, Pittman AW, Pulliam CC, et al. Renin profiling in hypertension and its use in treatment with propranolol and chlorthalidone. N Engl J Med. 1976;294:1137–1143.

12. Buhler FR, Bolli P, Kiowski W, et al. Renin profiling to select antihypertensive baseline drugs: Renin inhibitors for high-renin and calcium entry blockers for low-renin patients. Am J Med. 1984;77:36–42.

13. Letcher RL, Chien S, Laragh JH. Changes in blood viscosity accompanying the response to prazosin in patients with essential hypertension. J Cardiovasc Pharmacol. 1979;1(suppl 6):S8–S20.

14. Lund-Johansen P. Hemodynamic changes at rest and during exercise in long-term prazosin therapy for essential hypertension. In: Prazosin Clinical Symposium Proceedings. Special Proceedings by Postgraduate Medicine. New York: Custom Communications, McGraw-Hill Co, 1975:45–52.

15. Okun R. Effectiveness of prazosin as initial antihypertensive therapy. Am J Cardiol. 1983;51:644–650.

16. Itskovitz HD. Hemodynamic effects of antihypertensive drugs. Am Fam Physician. 1983;27:137–142.

17. van Zwieten PA, Thoolen MJ, Timmermans PB. The hypertensive activity and side effects of methyldopa, clonidine and guanfacine. Hypertension. 1984;6:1128–1133.

18. Lund-Johansen P. Hemodynamic changes in long-term diuretic therapy of essential hypertension: A comparative study of chlorthalidone, polythiazide and hydrochlorothiazide. Acta Med Scand. 1970;187:509–518.

19. Ventura HO, Frohlich ED, Messerli FH, et al. Immediate regional blood flow distribution following angiotensin converting enzyme inhibition in patients with essential hypertension. Am J Med. 1984;76:58–61.

20. Frohlich ED. Hemodynamic effects of calcium entry-blocking agents in normal and hypertensive rats and man. Am J Cardiol. 1985;56:21H–27H.

21. Halperin AK, Cubeddu LX. The role of calcium channel blockers in the treatment of hypertension. Am Heart J. 1986;111:363–382.

22. Ekelund LG, Ekelund C, Rossner S. Antihypertensive effects at rest and during exercise of a calcium blocker, nifedipine, alone and in combination with metoprolol. Acta Med Scand. 1982;212:71–75.

23. Lund-Johansen P. Hemodynamic effects of verapamil in essential hypertension at rest and during exercise. Acta Med Scand. 1984;681(suppl): 109–115.

24. Hansson L. Hemodynamics of metoprolol and pindolol in systemic hypertension with particular reference to reversal of structural vascular changes. Am J Cardiol. 1986;57:29C–32C.

25. Lund-Johansen P. Central hemodynamic effects of beta blockers in hypertension: A comparison between atenolol, metoprolol, timolol, penbutolol, alprenolol, pindolol and bunitrolol. Eur Heart J. 1983;4(suppl D): 1–12.

26. Trap-Jensen J, Clausen JP, Noer I, et al. The effects of beta-adrenoceptor blockers on cardiac output, liver blood flow and skeletal muscle blood flow in hypertensive patients. Acta Physiol Scand. 1976;440(suppl):30.

27. Pedersen EB. Abnormal renal hemodynamics during exercise in young patients with mild essential hypertension without treatment and during long-term propranolol therapy. Scand J Clin Lab Invest. 1978;30:567–571.

28. Hansson L, Pascual A, Julius S. Comparison of guanadrel and guanethidine. Clin Pharmacol Ther. 1973;14:204–208.

29. Woosley RL, Nies AS. Guanethidine. N Engl J Med. 1976;295: 1053–1057.

30. Lund-Johansen P. Exercise and antihypertensive therapy. Am J Cardiol. 1987;59:98A–107A.

31. Kannel WB, Wolf PA, Verter J, McNamara PM. Epidemiologic assessment of the role of blood pressure in stroke: The Framingham Study. JAMA. 1970;214:301–310.

32. Mortality Experience According to Blood Pressure After Treatment: Blood Pressure Study. Chicago: Society of Actuaries and Association of Life Insurance Medical Directors of America, 1979.

33. Hypertension Detection and Follow-up Program Cooperative Group. Five-year findings of the Hypertension Detection and Follow-Up Program: I. Reduction in mortality of persons with high blood pressure including mild hypertension. JAMA. 1979;242:2562–2571.

34. Veterans Administration Cooperative Study Group on Antihypertensive Agents. Effects of treatment on morbidity in hypertension: II. Results in patients with diastolic blood pressure averaging 90 through 114 mmHg. JAMA. 1970;213:1143–1152.

35. Smith WM. Treatment of mild hypertension: Results of a ten-year intervention trial. Circ Res. 1977;40(suppl I):198–205.

36. Perry HM Jr. Treatment of mild hypertension: Preliminary results of a two-year feasibility trial. Circ Res. 1977;40(suppl I):1180–1187.

37. Helgeland A. Treatment of mild hypertension: A five year controlled drug trial: The Oslo Study. Am J Med. 1980;69:725–732.

38. Report by the Management Committee: The Australian Therapeutic Trial in Mild Hypertension. Lancet. 1980;1:1261–1267.

39. Greenberg G, Brennan PJ, Miall WE. Effects of diuretic and beta-blocker therapy in the Medical Research Council Trial. Am J Med. 1984;76:45–51.

40. Multiple Risk Factor Intervention Trial Research Group. Multiple Risk Factor Intervention Trial: Risk factor changes and mortality results. JAMA. 1982;248:1465–1477.

41. Amery A, Birkenhäger W, Brixko P, et al. Mortality and morbidity results from the European Working Party on High Blood Pressure in the Elderly Trial. Lancet. 1985;1:1349–1354.

42. Miettinen TA, Huttunen JK, Naukkarinen V, et al. Multifactorial primary prevention of cardiovascular diseases in middle-aged men: Risk factor changes, incidence, and mortality. JAMA. 1985;254:2097–2102.

43. Wilhelmsen L, Tibblin G, Werkö L. A primary preventive study in Gothenburg, Sweden. Prev Med. 1972;1:153–160.

44. MRC Working Party. Medical Research Council trial of treatment of hypertension in older adults: Principal results. Br Med J. 1992;304:405–412.

45. U.S. Public Health Service Hospitals Cooperative Study Group, Smith WM. Treatment of mild hypertension: Results of a ten-year intervention trial. Circ Res. 1977;40(suppl I):I-98–I-105.

46. Perry HM Jr, Goldman AI, Lavin MA, et al. Evaluation of drug treatment in mild hypertension: VA-NHLBI feasibility trial. Ann NY Acad Sci. 1978;304:267–288.

47. IPPPSH Collaborative Group. Cardiovascular risk and risk factors in a randomized trial of treatment based on the beta-blocker oxprenolol: The International Prospective Primary Prevention Study in Hypertension (IPPPSH). J Hypertens. 1985;3:379–392.

48. Coope J, Warrender TS. Randomised trial of treatment of hypertension in elderly patients in primary care. Br Med J. 1986;293:1145–1151.

49. Wilhelmsen L, Berglund G, Elmfeldt D, et al. Beta-blockers versus diuretics in hypertensive men: Main results from the HAPPHY trial. J Hypertens. 1987;5:561–572.

50. Wikstrand J, Warnold I, Olsson G, et al. Primary prevention with metoprolol in patients with hypertension: Mortality results from the MAPHY study. JAMA. 1988;259:1976–1982.

51. SHEP Cooperative Research Group. Prevention of stroke by antihypertensive drug treatment in older persons with isolated systolic hypertension (SHEP): Final results of the Systolic Hypertension in the Elderly Program. JAMA. 1991;265:3255–3264.

52. Dahlöf B, Lindholm LH, Hansson L, et al. Morbidity and mortality in the Swedish Trial in Old Patients with Hypertension (STOP-Hypertension). Lancet. 1991;338:1281–1285.

53. Castelli WP. Epidemiology of coronary heart disease: The Framingham Study. Am J Med. 1984;76:4–12.

54. Castelli W, Leaf A. Identification and assessment of cardiac risk: An overview. Cardiol Clin. 1985;3:171–178.

55. Kannel WB. Status of risk factors and their consideration in antihypertensive therapy. Am J Cardiol. 1987;59:80A–90A.

56. Kannel WB, Schatzkin A. Risk factor analysis. Prog Cardiovasc Dis. 1983;26:309–332.

57. Bush TL, Barrett-Connor E, Cowan LD, et al. Cardiovascular mortality and noncontraceptive use of estrogen in women: Results from the Lipid Research Clinics Program Follow-Up Study. Circulation. 1987;75:1102–1109.

58. Deutsche RS. The effect of heavy drinking on ischemic heart disease. Primary Cardiol. 1986;12:40–48.

59. Fitzgerald DJ, Roy L, Catella F, Fitzgerald GA. Platelet activation in unstable coronary disease. N Engl J Med 1986;315:983–989.

60. Meade TW, Mellows S, Brozovic M, et al. Haemostatic function and ischaemic heart disease: Principal results of the Northwick Park Heart Study. Lancet. 1986;2:533–537.

61. Spence JD. Hemodynamic effects of antihypertensive drugs: Possible implications for the prevention of atherosclerosis. Hypertension. 1984; 6:163–168.

62. Brunner HR, Laragh JH, Baer L, et al. Essential hypertension: Renin and aldosterone, heart attack and stroke. N Engl J Med. 1972;286:441–449.

63. Giese J. Renin, angiotensin and hypertensive vascular damage: A review. Am J Med. 1973;55:315–332.

64. Chobanian AV. The influence of hypertension and other hemodynamic factors in atherogenesis. Prog Cardiovasc Dis. 1983;26:177–196.

65. Letcher RL, Chien S, Pickering TG, et al. Direct relationship between blood pressure and blood viscosity in normal and hypertensive subjects: Role of fibrinogen and concentration. Am J Med. 1981;70:1195–1202.

66. Reaven GM, Huffman BB. A role for insulin in the aetiology and course of hypertension. Lancet. 1987;2:435–437.

67. Ferrannini E, Buzzigoli G, Bonadonna R, et al. Insulin resistance in essential hypertension. N Engl J Med. 1987;317:435–437.

68. Ames RP, Hill P. Elevation of serum lipid levels during diuretic therapy of hypertension. Am J Med. 1976;61:748–757.

69. Lasser NL, Grandits G, Caggiula AW, et al. Effects of antihypertensive therapy on plasma lipids and lipoproteins in the Multiple Risk Factor Intervention Trial. Am J Med. 1984;76:52–66.

70. Helgeland A, Hjermann L, Leren P, Holme I. Possible metabolic side effects of beta-adrenergic blocking drugs. Br Med J. 1978;1:828.

71. Ames RP. The effects of antihypertensive drugs on serum lipids and lipoproteins: I. Diuretics. Drugs. 1986;32:260–278.

72. Ames RP, Hill P. Increase in serum lipids during treatment of hypertension with chlorthalidone. Lancet. 1976;1:721–723.

73. Glück Z, Weidmann P, Mordasini R, et al. Increased serum low-density lipoprotein cholesterol in men treated short-term with the diuretic chlorthalidone. Metabolism. 1980;29:240–245.

74. Boehringer K, Weidmann P, Mordasini R, et al. Menopause-dependent plasma lipoprotein alterations in diuretic-treated women. Ann Intern Med. 1982;97:206–209.

75. Mauersberger H. Effect of prazosin on blood pressure and plasma lipids in patients receiving a beta-blocker and diuretic regimen. Am J Med. 1984;76:101–104.

76. Goldman AI, Steele BW, Schnaper HW, et al. Serum lipoprotein levels during chlorthalidone therapy: A Veterans Administration–National Heart, Lung, and Blood Institute cooperative study on antihypertensive therapy: Mild hypertension. JAMA. 1980;224:1691–1695.

77. Koskinen P, Manninen V, Eisalo A. Quinapril and blood lipids. Br J Clin Pharmacol. 1988;26:478–480.

78. Ames RP. Metabolic disturbances increasing the risk of coronary heart disease during diuretic-based antihypertensive therapy: Lipid alterations and glucose intolerance. Am Heart J. 1983;106:1207–1214.

79. Ames RP. Negative effects of diuretic drugs on metabolic risk factors for coronary heart disease: Possible alternative drug therapies. Am J Cardiol. 1983;51:632–638.

80. Grimm RH Jr, Leon AS, Hunninghake DB, et al. Effects of thiazide diuretics on plasma lipids and lipoproteins in mildly hypertensive patients: A double-blind controlled trial. Ann Intern Med. 1981;94:7–11.

81. Flamenbaum W. Metabolic consequences of antihypertensive therapy. Ann Intern Med. 1983;98:875–880.

82. Weinberger MH. Antihypertensive therapy and lipids: Evidence, mechanisms, and implications. Arch Intern Med. 1985;145:1102–1105.

83. Drayer JI, Gardin JM, Weber MA, Aronow WS. Changes in ventricular septal thickness during diuretic therapy. Clin Pharmacol Ther. 1982; 32:283–288.

84. Lowenthal DT. Hypertension and exercise physiology: Clinical and therapeutic applications. In: Lowenthal DT, Bharadwaja K, Oaks WW, eds. Therapeutics Through Exercise. New York: Grune & Stratton, 1981:133–144.

85. Loaldi A, Polese A, Montorsi P, et al. Comparison of nifedipine, propranolol and isosorbide dinitrate on angiographic progression and regression of coronary arterial narrowings in angina pectoris. Am J Cardiol. 1989;64:433–439.

86. Lichtlen PR, Hugenholtz PG, Rafflenbeul W, et al. Retardation of angiographic progression of coronary artery disease by nifedipine: Results of the International Nifedipine Trial on Antiatherosclerotic Therapy (INTACT). Lancet. 1990;335:1109–1113.

87. Kober G, Schneider W, Kaltenbach M. Can the progression of coronary sclerosis be influenced by calcium antagonists? J Cardiovasc Pharmacol. 1989;13(suppl 4):52–56.

88. The MIDAS Research Group. Multicenter Isradipine Diuretic Atherosclerosis Study (MIDAS). Am J Med. 1989;86(suppl 4A):37–39.

89. Waters D, Lespérance J. Interventions that beneficially influence the evolution of coronary atherosclerosis: The case for calcium channel blockers. Circulation. 1992;86(suppl III):III-111–III-116.

90. Rostand SG, Brown G, Kirk KA, et al. Renal insufficiency in treated essential hypertension. N Engl J Med. 1989;320:684–688.

91. Brazy PC, Fitzwilliam JF. Progressive renal disease: Role of race and antihypertensive medications. Kidney Int. 1990;37:1113–1119.

92. Eliahou HE, Cohen D, Hellberg B, et al. Effect of the calcium channel blocker nisoldipine on the progression of chronic renal failure in man. Am J Nephrol. 1988;8:285–290.

93. Alcazar JM, Rodicio JL, Ruilope LM. Long-term diuretic therapy and renal function in essential arterial hypertension. Am J Cardiol. 1990; 65:51H–54H.

94. Warram JH, Laffel LMB, Valsania P, et al. Excess mortality associated with diuretic therapy in diabetes mellitus. Arch Intern Med. 1991; 151:1350 1356.

95. Croog SH, Levine S, Testa MA, et al. The effects of antihypertensive therapy on the quality of life. N Engl J Med. 1986;314:1657–1664.

96. Jachuck SJ, Brierly J, Jachuck S, Willcox PM. The effect of hypotensive drugs on the quality of life. J R Coll Gen Pract. 1982;32:103–105.

97. Curb JD, Borhani NO, Blaszkowski TP, et al. Long-term surveillance for adverse effects of antihypertensive drugs. JAMA. 1985;253:3263–3268.

98. Avorn J, Everitt DE, Weiss S. Increased antidepressant use in patients prescribed β-blockers. JAMA. 1986;255;357–360.

99. Testa MA, Hollenberg HK, Anderson RB, Williams GH. Assessment of quality of life by patient and spouse during antihypertensive therapy with atenolol and nifedipine gastrointestinal therapeutic system. Am J Hypertens. 1991;4:363–373.

100. Os I, Bratland B, Dahløf B, et al. Lisinopril or nifedipine in essential hypertension? A Norwegian multicenter study on efficacy, tolerability and quality of life in 828 patients. J Hypertens. 1991;9:1097–1104.

101. Croog SH, Kong BW, Levine S, et al. Hypertensive black men and women. Quality of life and effects of antihypertensive medications. Arch Intern Med. 1990;150:1733–1741.

102. Fletcher AE, Bulpitt CJ, Hawkins CM, et al. Quality of life on antihypertensive therapy: a randomized double-blind controlled trial of captopril and atenolol. J Hypertens. 1990;8:463–466.

103. Gerber JC, Nies AS. Pharmacology of antihypertensive drugs. In: Genest J, Kuchel O, Hamet P, et al. Hypertension. 2nd ed. New York, NY: McGraw-Hill; 1983:1093 1127.

104. Wollam GL, Gifford RW, Tarazi RC. Antihypertensive drugs. Clin Pharmacol Ther Drugs. 1977;14:420–460.

105. Carney S, Gillies Al, Morgan T. Optimal dose of a thiazide diuretic. Med J Aust. 1976;2:692–693.

106. Campbell DB, Brackman F. Cardiovascular protective properties of indapamide. Am J Cardiol. 1990;65:11H–27H.

107. Clarke RJ. Indapamide: A diuretic of choice for the treatment of hypertension? Am J Med Sci. 1991;301(3):215–220.

108. Oster JR, Epstein M. Use of centrally acting sympatholytic agents in the management of hypertension. Arch Intern Med. 1991;151:1638–1644.

109. Beers MH, Passman LJ. Antihypertensive medications and depression. Drugs. 1990;40(6):792–799.

110. Ames RP. The effects of antihypertensive drugs on serum lipids and lipoproteins. Part II. Non-diuretic drugs. Drugs. 1986;32:335–357.

111. Kaplan NM. Resistant hypertension: What to do after trying "the usual." Geriatrics. 1995;50:24–38.

112. Houston MC. Pathophysiology, clinical aspects diagnosis and treatment of hypertensive crisis. Prog Cardiovasc Dis. 1989;32:99–148.

113. Cunningham FG, Lindheimer H. Hypertension in pregnancy. N Engl J Med. 1992;326:927–932.

114. Sabatini S. Pathophysiology of and therapeutic strategies for hypertension in pregnancy. Curr Opin Nephrol Hypertens. 1993;2:763–774.

115. Kincaid-Smith, P. Hypertension in pregnancy. Blood Pressure. 1994;3:18–23.

116. Joint National Committee on Prevention, Detection, Evaluation, and Treatment of High Blood Pressure. The Sixth Report of the Joint National Committee on Prevention, Detection, Evaluation, and Treatment of High Blood Pressure. Arch Intern Med. 1997;157:2413–2446.

117. Hilleman DE, Mohiuddin SM, Lucas D Jr, et al. Cost-minimization analysis of initial antihypertensive therapy in patients with mild to moderate essential diastolic hypertension (ABST). Circulation 1992;88(Part 2):263.

118. Himmelmann, A, Hansson L, et al. ACE inhibition prescribes renal function better than beta-blockade in the treatment of essential hypertension. Blood Pressure. 1995;4:85–90.

119. Saruta T, Kanns Y, et al. Renal effects of amlodipine. J Hum Hypertens. 1995;9(suppl I):811–816.

120. Reeves RA. Does this patient have hypertension? How to measure blood pressure. JAMA. 1995;273:1211–1218.

121. Drugs for Hypertension. Med Lett. 1995;37:45–50.

122. Eberhardt RT, Kevak RM, Kang PM, Frishman WH. Angiotensin II receptor blockade: An innovative approach to cardiovascular pharmacotherapy. J Clin Pharmacol. 1993;33:1023–1038.

123. Gradman AH, Arcuri KE, Goldberg AI, et al. A randomized, placebo-controlled, double-blind, parallel study of various doses of losartan potassium compared with enalapril maleate in patients with essential hypertension. Hypertension. 1995;25:1345–1350.

124. Bakris, GL, Griffen KA. Combined effects of an angiotensin converting enzyme inhibitor and a calcium antagonist on renal injury. J Hypertens. 1997;15:1181–1185.

125. Bakris GL, Houston MC, Messerli FH. Effective use of combination therapy in hypertension. Patient Care. Fall 1997 suppl., pp 10–21.

126. Gong L, Zhang W. Shanghai Trial of Nifedipine in the Elderly (STONE). J Hypertens. 1996;14:1237–1245.

127. Staessen J. Facard R. et al. Systolic Hypertension in Europe Trial (SYST–EUR). Lancet. 1997;350:757–764.

128. Liu L, Wang JG, Gong L, et al. Comparison of active treatment and placebo in older Chinese patients with isolated systolic hypertension: Systolic Hypertension in China (Syst-China) Collaborative Group. J Hypertens. 1998;16:1823–1829.

129. Hansson L. Zanchetti A, Carruthers SG, et al. Effects of intensive blood pressure lowering and low-dose aspirin in patients with hypertension: Principal results of the Hypertension Optimal Treatment (HOT) randomized trial. Lancet. 1998;351:1755–1762.

130. Messerli FH, Grossman E, Goldbourt U. Are beta-blockers efficacious as first-line therapy for hypertension in the elderly? A systematic review. JAMA. 1998;279:1903–1907.

131. Bakris GL. Progression of diabetic nephropathy: A focus on arterial pressure level and methods of reduction. Diabetes Res Clin Pract. 1998;39(Suppl):S35–S42.

132. Epstein M. The benefits of ACE inhibitors and calcium antagonists in slowing progressive renal failure: Focus on fixed-dose combination antihypertensive therapy. Ren Fail. 1996;18:813–832.

133. Hansson L, Lindholm LH, Niskanen L, et al. Effect of angiotensin-converting enzyme inhibition compared with conventional therapy on cardiovascular morbidity and mortality in hypertension: The Captopril Prevention Project (CAPPP). Lancet. 1999;611–616.

134. Tuomilehto J, Rastenyte D, Birkenhäger W, et al. Effects of calcium-channel blockade in older patients with diabetes and systolic hypertension. N Engl J Med 1999;340:677-684.

135. National Intervention Cooperative Study in Elderly Hypertensives Study Group: Randomized double-blind comparison of a calcium antagonist and a diuretic in elderly hypertensives. Hypertension 1999;34:1129-1133.

136. Hansson L, Lindholm LH, Ekbom T, et al, for the STOP-Hypertension-2 Study Group: Randomized trial of old and new antihypertensive drugs in elderly patients: Cardiovascular mortality and morbidity the Swedish Trial in Old Patients with Hypertension-2 study. Lancet 1999;354:1751-1756.

137. US Renal Data System: USRDS 1997 Annual Data Report. Bethesda, MD, National Institute of Health, National Institute of Diabetes and Digestive and Kidney Diseases, 1997.

138. Klag MJ, Whelton PK et al: Blood pressure and incidence of end stage renal disease in men. A prospective study. Circulation 1994; 18:941.

139. National High Blood Pressure Education Program Working Group: 1995 update of the working group reports on chronic renal failure and renovascular hypertension. Arch Int. Med 1996;156:1938-1947.

140. Bauer JH, Reams GP, Lai SM: Renal protective effects of strict blood pressure control with enalapril therapy. Arch Intern Med 1987;147:1387-1400.

141. Wee PM, De Mitchell AG, Epstein M: Effects of calcium antagonists on renal hemodynamics and progression of nondiabetic chronic renal disease. Arch Intern Med 1994;154:1185-1202.

142. Hannedouche T, Landais P, et al: Randomised controlled trial of enalapril and beta-blockers in non-diabetic chronic renal failure. BMJ 1994;309:833-837.

143. GISEN Study Group: Randomized placebo controlled trial of the effect of ramipiril on decline in glomerular filtration rate and risk of terminal renal failure in proteinuric nondiabetic nephropathy. Lancet 1997; 349:1857-1863.

144. Maschio G, Alberti D, Hanin G, et al: Effect of the angiotensin-converting enzyme inhibitor benazapril on the progression of renal insufficiency. N Engl J Med 1996;334:939-945.

145. Tarif N, Bakris GL: Angiotensin II receptor blockade and progression of renal disease in non-diabetic patients. Kidney Int 1997;52(Suppl 63):S-67-S-70.

146. Bakris GL (ed): The renin-angiotensin system in diabetic nephropathy: From bench to bedside. Miner Electrolyte Metab 1998; 24(6):361-438.

147. Neutel JM, Smith DHG, Weber MA: Is high blood pressure a late manifestation of the hypertension syndrome? Am J Hypertens 1999; 12:215S-223S.

148. Messerli FH, Grossman E: B-blockers and diuretics: to use or not to use? Am J Hypertens 1999;12:157S-163S.

149. Abernethy, DR, Schwartz JB: Calcium antagonist drugs. N Engl J Med 1999; 341(19):1447-1457.